Molecular Diagnostics

Molecular Diagnostics

A Training and Study Guide

Gregory J. Tsongalis, PhD
Department of Pathology and Laboratory Medicine
Hartford Hospital
Hartford, Connecticut

and

William B. Coleman, PhD
Department of Pathology and Laboratory Medicine
University of North Carolina School of Medicine
Chapel Hill, North Carolina

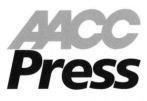

2101 L Street, NW, Suite 202
Washington, DDC 20037-1558

1 2 3 4 5 6 7 8 9 0   GG   03   02   01

Printed in the United States of America

Library of Congress Cataloging-in-Publication Data

Tsongalis, Gregory J.
    Molecular diagnostics : a training and study guide / Gregory J. Tsongalis and William B. Coleman.
        p. ; cm.
    ISBN 1-890883-76-X (alk. paper)
    1. Molecular diagnosis. 2. Pathology, Molecular. I. Coleman, William B. II. Title.
    [DNLM: 1. Molecular Diagnostic Techniques—methods—Examination Questions. QZ 18.2 T882m 2002]
RB43.7 .T76 2002
616.07′56—dc21

2002066719

Contents

Foreword

The rapidly developing field of molecular diagnostics encompasses the application of sequence-based information to the clinical laboratory environment in three converging areas: (1) information derived from the Human Genome Project regarding genomic organization; (2) the association of genomic sequence data with health and disease; and (3) the development of sophisticated and reliable technologies. Although considerable work remains to be done in each of these areas, the immediate challenge is to educate health care professionals and provide training programs for the molecular personnel who will be performing and interpreting these exciting new diagnostic tests.

Molecular Diagnosis: A Training and Study Guide serves as a primer for both laboratorians and educators. In the laboratory setting, new information regarding inherited disorders, identity testing, infectious diseases, and oncology translates into useful clinical data. It is for this reason that we must introduce current molecular diagnostics information to medical students, residents, fellows, graduate students, and clinical laboratory technologists. This formidable task is approached systematically in this study and training guide. Background information is provided in the first eight chapters, with specific applications comprising the next five chapters. Finally, a comprehensive self-assessment section provides feedback to the reader.

Obviously, with changes occurring rapidly in molecular diagnostics, no printed material can be completely current. For laboratorians and educators alike, laboratory medicine will never be the same. However, this guide can provide a firm foundation for the ambitious reader entering the twenty-first century.

Lawrence M. Silverman, Ph.D.   February 6, 2002
University of North Carolina
Chapel Hill, North Carolina

Introduction

Molecular Diagnostics: A Training and Study Guide represents a compilation of educational materials we have assembled over several years of academic instruction at the undergraduate and graduate levels. Given the increasing numbers of board certification exams that have emerged for this discipine over this time period, we hope that this manuscript will function as a guide for development of training/review courses and study preparation. By no means have we intended this manuscript to be comprehensive of all molecular biology, but it should serve as an excellent overview of those technologies most pertinent to clinical diagnostic applications. This guide contains thirteen sections covering human genome efforts, basic molecular biology concepts, a review of technology, issues in diagnostic testing, and finally, clinical applications in various disciplines of laboratory medicine. In addition, we have included an extensive self-assessment section that covers much of the material presented.

It is our intention that this guide serve to educate, train, and promote the field of molecular diagnostics to all who are willing to learn.

Gregory J. Tsongalis
William B. Coleman

SECTION 1

Introduction to Molecular Diagnostics

_____

_____

_____

_____

_____

_____

_____

Goal

To introduce essential concepts in molecular diagnostics that impact on the identification of novel markers of human diseases and to develop and apply useful molecular assays to monitor disease, determine appropriate treatment strategies, and predict disease outcomes.

_____

_____

_____

_____

_____

_____

Outline

- Definition of molecular diagnostics
- Impact of molecular diagnostics in human disease
- Molecular pathology in laboratory medicine
- Molecular biology timeline
- Genomic technologies and applications
- Future prospects for molecular diagnostics

_____

_____

_____

_____

_____

_____

Molecular Diagnostics

The use of molecular biology techniques to expand scientific knowledge of the natural history of diseases, identify people who are at risk for acquiring specific diseases, and diagnose infectious and other human diseases at the nucleic acid level.

**Guiding Principles for the Discovery
of Novel Molecular Markers
of Human Disease**

Identification of novel molecular markers of
human disease will facilitate the development
of useful molecular assays for detection,
diagnosis, and prediction of disease outcomes.

Molecular Diagnostics

- Monitor diseases more accurately
  - Allows for early treatment and better patient
    care
- Determine most appropriate treatment
  - Reduces or eliminates unnecessary
    treatment
  - Reduces or eliminates inadequate treatment
  - Yields greater cost effectiveness
- Reduce patient morbidity and mortality

**Practical Applications of Molecular
Diagnostics in Laboratory Medicine**

- Diagnostic
- Prognostic
- Therapeutic
- Predictive

_____

_____

_____

_____

_____

_____

_____

_____

_____

_____

_____

_____

_____

_____

_____

_____

_____

_____

_____

_____

_____

Applications of Genomic Technologies in Laboratory Medicine

- Anatomic pathology
- Chemistry/toxicology
- Genetics
- Hematopathology/oncology
- Infectious diseases
- Transfusion medicine/identity

Molecular Pathology
A Universal Discipline of Laboratory Medicine

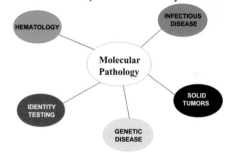

Practical Applications of Molecular Diagnostics in Clinical Laboratory Medicine

Molecular Genetics
- Single gene disorders
- Polygenic disorders
- Chromosomal disorders

Molecular Oncology
- Diagnostic testing
- Disease prognosis
- Determination of predisposition

**Practical Applications of
Molecular Diagnostics in
Clinical Laboratory Medicine** *(cont.)*

Hematopathology
- Diagnostic testing
- Determination of clonality

Identity Testing
- Parentage
- Clinical testing

**Practical Applications of
Molecular Diagnostics in
Clinical Laboratory Medicine** *(cont.)*

Infectious Disease
- Qualitative and quantitative detection of infectious agents
- Microbial identity testing
- Genotyping/drug resistance testing

Advances in the understanding of the structure and chemistry of nucleic acids have facilitated the development of technologies that can be employed effectively in molecular diagnostics.

_____

_____

_____

_____

_____

_____

_____

The Molecular Biology Timeline

1865	Gregor Mendel, Law of Heredity
1866	Johann Miescher, Purification of DNA
1953	Watson and Crick, Structure of DNA
1970	Recombinant DNA Technology
1977	Sickle Cell Anemia Mutation
1980	_In Vitro_ Amplification of DNA (PCR)
1995	The Human Genome Project

_____

_____

_____

_____

_____

Molecular Technologies in the Clinical Laboratory

Blotting Techniques   **Electrophoretic Methods**
Southern hybridization   SSCP
Northern hybridization   DGGE MDE

Amplification Techniques
PCR   TMA
LCR   NASBA
bDNA

DNA Sequencing

_____

_____

_____

_____

_____

_____

Why are Nucleic Acids Important in the Clinical Laboratory?

• Genetically-based diseases can be diagnosed.

• Specificity can be controlled.

• Single base changes can be detected.

• Expression of gene product is not required.

• Targets can be amplified $>10^5$.

Human Disease

Cause (etiology)

↓

Mechanism (pathogenesis)

↓

Structural alterations (morphologic/molecular)

↓

Functional consequences (clinical significance)

**Understanding the Molecular
Pathogenesis of Human Disease
Enables Effective Utilization of
Molecular Assays**

Diagnostic
- Distinguishing variants of human disease based on presence of specific molecular markers (chromosome translocations in lymphoma)

Prognostic
- Prediction of likely patient outcomes based on presence of specific molecular markers (gene mutations predicting poor clinical course in cancer)

**Understanding the Molecular
Pathogenesis of Human Disease
Enables Effective Utilization of
Molecular Assays** *(cont.)*

Therapeutic
- Prediction of response to specific therapies based on presence of specific molecular markers (gene mutations predicting poor drug sensitivity in cancer)

_____

_____

_____

_____

_____

_____

_____

_____

_____

_____

_____

_____

_____

_____

_____

_____

_____

Future Prospects
for Molecular Diagnostics

Continued advances in the understanding of the molecular basis of human disease will facilitate development of new and useful molecular diagnostics for a range of human disease conditions.

Ultimately, identification of disease-causing genes and/or genes that modify disease expression or response to treatment will expand the number of molecular diagnostics applications that will be required for the basic clinical workup of patients.

The Molecular Basis
of Human Disease

Genetic Lesions in Human Disease
- Identification of genetic markers
- Identification of disease-related genes
- Molecular targets for assay development

Characterization of Gene Sequences
- Facilitates characterization of disease-causing mutations
- Molecular targets for assay development

The Molecular Basis
of Human Disease _(cont.)_

Completion of the sequence of the human genome will enable identification of all human genes and establishment of disease-gene relationships, facilitating development of numerous new molecular assays.

The Human Genome Project

- U.S. Government project coordinated by the Department of Energy and the National Institutes of Health
- Goals of the Human Genome Project (1998–2003)
  - to identify all of the genes in human DNA;
  - to determine the sequences of the 3 billion bases that make up human DNA;
  - to create databases;
  - to develop tools for data analysis; and
  - to address the ethical, legal, and social issues that arise from genome research.

Beneficial Outcomes from the Human Genome Project

- Improvements in medicine
- Microbial genome research
- DNA forensics/identity
- Improved agriculture and livestock
- Better understanding of evolution and human migration
- More accurate risk assessment

The Human Genome Project
Ethical, Legal, and Social Implications

- Use of genetic information
- Privacy/confidentiality
- Psychological impact and stigmatization
- Genetic testing
- Reproductive options/issues
- Education, standards, and quality control
- Commercialization
- Conceptual and philosophical implications

_____

_____

_____

_____

_____

_____

_____

Molecular Diagnostics in Clinical Practice

The ultimate goal of the molecular diagnostics laboratory is to provide molecular information that will combine with and complement information related to patient history and symptomology, clinical laboratory results, histopathological findings, and other diagnostic information to provide a more sensitive, precise, and accurate determination of disease diagnosis and/or guidance toward appropriate and effective treatment options.

Biochemistry and Organization of the Human Genome

_____

_____

_____

_____

_____

_____

_____

Goal

To describe the chemistry, structure, and function of nucleic acids, including essential concepts of genetic variation, gene and chromosome structure, and DNA sequence.

_____

_____

_____

_____

_____

_____

_____

Outline

- Molecular structure of DNA
- Chemical composition of DNA
- Functional units of DNA
- Genetic variation
- The Human Genome Project

_____

_____

_____

_____

_____

_____

_____

The Discovery of the Structure of DNA

J.D. Watson and F.H.C. Crick (1953)
A structure for deoxyribose nucleic acid.
Nature 171:737

"We wish to suggest a structure for the salt of deoxyribose nucleic acid (D.N.A.). This structure has novel features which are of considerable biological interest."

The Discovery of the Structure of DNA

Rosalind E. Franklin
1920–1958

The structure of DNA was determined using X-ray diffraction techniques. Much of the original X-ray diffraction data was generated by Rosalind E. Franklin.

The Structure of DNA

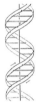

The original structure of DNA proposed by Watson and Crick in their 1953 paper (*Nature* 171:737)

1962 Nobel Prize for Medicine

"... for their discoveries concerning the molecular structure of nucleic acids and its significance for information transfer in living material ..."

J.D. Watson   F.H.C. Crick   M.H.F. Wilkins

_____

_____

_____

_____

_____

_____

_____

DNA—The Chemical Basis of Heredity

- Biological "blueprint"
  - Carries information for cells to live, grow, differentiate, and replicate
  - Provides consistency and variability

_____

_____

_____

_____

_____

_____

Human DNA

- Diploid genome (two sets of chromosomes)
- Packaged in 23 pairs of chromosomes
- 22 homologous pairs (autosomes)
- 2 sex chromosomes (XX or XY)
- 6 billion bases
- 50,000–100,000 genes

_____

_____

_____

_____

_____

_____

The Human Chromosome

- Single linear duplex DNA
- Numerous protein interactions
- DNA from a single cell measures approximately 2 meters in length
- Histones → Nucleosomes → Solenoids

Human DNA

- Less than 10% codes for protein

- Heterochromatin: densely packed region of chromosomes (centromeres), not transcribed

- Euchromatin: less densely packed, transcribed regions

- Approximately 75% of the genome is unique or single copy

DNA Structure

- Consists of a pair of antiparallel strands $(5' \rightarrow 3'$ and $3' \rightarrow 5')$
- Alternating deoxyribose and phosphate groups
- Covalent linkage by phosphodiester bonds
- Strands held together by hydrogen bonds

DNA Structure

- Linked sequences of nucleotides
- Nucleotides consist of a nitrogenous base, five carbon sugar, and a phosphate group
- Sequence of bases determines genetic information

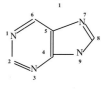

Components of DNA Structure
Nitrogenous Bases

- **Pyrimidines**
  - 6-member ring
  - cytosine, thymine, uracil
- **Purines**
  - fused 5- and 6-member rings
  - adenine, guanine

Nitrogenous Bases

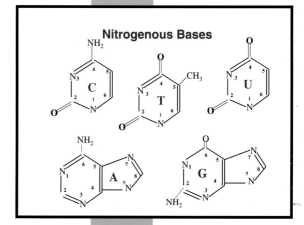

Pentose Sugars

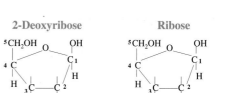

Polynucleotide Chain

Nucleotide base

Sugar-phosphate backbone

The Building Blocks of DNA

Nucleoside = base + sugar

Nucleotide = base + sugar + phosphate

DNA Structure

- Adenine binds Thymine (A:T).
- Guanine binds Cytosine (G:C).
- G:C pair contains three hydrogen bonds.
- A:T pair contains two hydrogen bonds.
- Complementarity refers to this unique base-pair matching in the structure of DNA.
- Polarity describes the orientation of the DNA strand with reference to the 5′-phosphate and 3′-hydroxyl groups.

DNA Structure

Denaturation of DNA describes the separation of the duplex strands through one of several conditions:

– Alkaline pH

– Strong hydrogen bond solvents

– Elevated temperature

DNA Structure

DNA melting temperature (T_m) is the temperature at which 50% of dsDNA denatures to give ssDNA. Determination of T_m depends on several factors:
- G:C content of the DNA
- length of dsDNA
- ionic strength of the solution
- pH of the solution
- the presence of hydrogen bond solvents, such as formamide
- the number of base-pair mismatches

DNA Structure

Phosphate–Sugar Backbone
- Acidic (pKa 2–4)
- Negatively charged
- Polar soluble
- Migrates to anode (+)
- Links nucleotides in ssDNA
- Binds cations

Purine/Pyrimidine Bases
- Alkaline (pKa 8–10)
- Uncharged
- Organic soluble
- Determines amino acid sequence
- Holds duplex DNA strands together by hydrogen bonding
- Binds intercalating agents

Genetic Units of DNA

Nuclear DNA

- 22 autosomes
- 2 sex (X,Y) chromosomes
- 120 million bases per chromosome
- 50,000–100,00 genes

Mitochondrial DNA

- 16,569 base pairs
- 37 genes
- Higher mutation rate
- 128 naturally occurring polymorphisms
- Maternal inheritance

Genetic Units of DNA Encoded in Mitochondrial DNA

- Ribosomal RNA (16S, 22S)
- 22 mitochondrial tRNAs
- 7 subunits of respiratory complex I (NADH-Ubiquinol Oxidoreductase)
- 1 subunit of respiratory complex III (Ubiquinol-Cytochrome C Oxidoreductase)
- 3 subunits of respiratory complex IV (Cytochrome C Oxidase)
- 2 subunits of respiratory complex V (ATP Synthase)

RNA Structure

- Single-stranded
- Ribose sugar substituted for deoxyribose of DNA
- Uracil replaces thymine of DNA
- A:U (uracil)

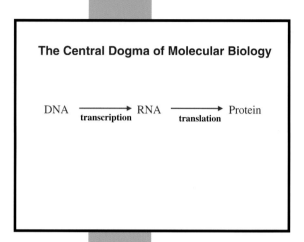

The Central Dogma of Molecular Biology

DNA $\xrightarrow{\text{transcription}}$ RNA $\xrightarrow{\text{translation}}$ Protein

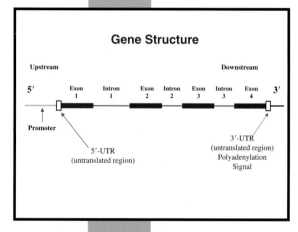

Gene Structure

Upstream

Downstream

5′ Exon 1 Intron 1 Exon 2 Intron 2 Exon 3 Intron 3 Exon 4 3′

Promoter

5′-UTR
(untranslated region)

3′-UTR
(untranslated region)
Polyadenylation
Signal

Types of Genetic Variants

- Structural
  - Gain/loss of chromosome segments
  - Translocations
  - Rearrangements
  - Gene amplifications
- Molecular
  - Deletions/insertions
  - Nucleotide repeats (di-, tri-)
  - Point mutations (RFLPs, SNPs)

The Human Genome

```
  1 ctccgggctg tcccagctcg gcaagcgctg cccaggtcct ggggtggtgg cagccagcgg
 61 gagcaggaaa ggaagcatgt tcccaggctg cccacgcctc tgggtcctgg tggtcttggg
121 caccagctgg gtaggctggg ggagccaagg gacagaagcg gcacagctaa ggcagttcta
181 cgtggctgct cagggcatca gttggagcta ccgacctgag cccacaaact caagtttgaa
241 tctttctgta acttccttta agaaaattgt ctacagagag tatgaaccat attttaagaa
301 agaaaaacca caatctacca tttcaggact tcttgggcct actttatatg ctgaagtcgg
361 agacatcata aaagttcact ttaaaaataa ggcagataag cccttgagca tccatcctca
421 aggaattagg tacagtaaat tatcagaagg tgcttcttac cttgaccaca cattccctgc
481 agagaagatg gacgacgctg tggctccagg ccgagaatac acctatgaat ggagtatcag
541 tgaggacagt ggacccaccc atgatgaccc tccatgcctc acacacatct attactccca
601 tgaaaatctg atcgaggatt tcaactctgg gctgattggg cccctgctta tctgtaaaaa
661 agggaccccta actgagggtg ggacacagaa gacgtttgac aagcaaatcg tgctactatt
721 tgctgtgttt gatgaaagca agagctggag ccagtcatca tccctaatgt acacagtcaa
781 tggatatgtg aatgggacaa tgccagatat aacagtttgt gcccatgacc acatcagctg
841 gcatctgctg ggaatgagct cggggccaga atattctcc attcatttca acggccaggt
901 cctggagcag aaccatcata aggtctcagc catcacccct gtcagtgcta catccactac
961 cgcaaatatg actgtgggcc cagagggaaa gtggatcata tcttctctca ccccaaaaca
```

Human Diseases

Cause (etiology)

↓

Mechanism (pathogenesis)

↓

Structural alterations (morphologic/molecular)

↓

Functional consequences (clinical significance)

Specimen Collection, Handling, Preparation, and Processing

Goal

To introduce essential concepts and fundamentals of collection and handling of clinical specimens for the molecular diagnostics laboratory, to describe basic methods of DNA and RNA isolation, and to introduce methods used in the analysis of DNA and RNA.

Outline

- Principles for handling clinical specimens
- Types of specimens
- Fundamentals of specimen handling
- Nucleic acid preparation
- DNA isolation methods
- RNA isolation methods
- Methods of analysis of nucleic acids

Principles for Handling of All Clinical Specimens

- Observe universal precautions for biohazards.
- Use protective gowns, gloves, face and eye shields.
- Decontaminate all spills and work areas with 10% bleach.
- Dispose of all waste in appropriate biologic waste containers.
- Use gloves. Your RNA depends on it!

Types of Specimens for the Molecular Diagnostics Laboratory

- Whole blood
- Bone marrow
- PBSC (phoresis product)
- Serum/plasma
- Buccal cells
- Cultured cells
- Blood spots

- Body fluids
  – CSF
  – Bronchial lavage
  – Amniotic
  – Semen
  – Urine
- Tissue samples
  – Fresh/frozen
  – Paraffin-embedded
- Hair (shaft/root)

Fundamentals of Specimen Handling
Specimen Labeling

- Patient name, date of birth, and medical record number
- Ordering physician
- Type of specimen
- Accession number
- Date and time of collection
- Laboratory technician identification (initials)
- Requested test(s)

Blood and Bone Marrow

- Isolation of nucleic acids (genomic DNA or RNA)

- Collection: Collect in an anticoagulant, mix well but gently to avoid disruption of cells

---

Anticoagulants

EDTA
- Lavender-top Vacutainer
- Preferred specimen

ACD
- Yellow-top Vacutainer

Heparin
- Green-top Vacutainer
- Inhibits several enzymes used in molecular assays

Specimen Packaging and Shipping
Blood and Bone Marrow

- **DO NOT FREEZE!!!**
- Protect from temperature extremes
- Overnight delivery preferred
- Packaging must comply with shipping rules for bloodborne pathogens
  - Protective container
  - Absorbent material in packing
  - Sealed container in plastic bag
  - Labeled as **Biohazard**

Paraffin-embedded Tissue Sections

- Genetic testing, infectious disease testing, identity testing
- Formalin-fixed tissue is suitable.
- Mercury or other heavy metal fixatives are not acceptable.
- Tissue sections on glass slides can be used for *in situ* applications and microdissection techniques.

Specimen Storage Requirements—DNA

Blood, Bone Marrow, Other Fluids

- 22–25 °C Not recommended ($\leq$24 hours)
- 2–8 °C   Suitable condition for up to 72 hours
- –20 °C   Not recommended
  - **NOTE**: Do not freeze blood or bone marrow before lysing red blood cells (RBCs). Leukocyte pellet can be frozen for up to 1 year.
- –70 °C   Not recommended
  - **NOTE**: Do not freeze blood or bone marrow before lysing red blood cells (RBCs). Leukocyte pellet can be frozen for >1 year.

Specimen Storage Requirements — RNA

Blood, Bone Marrow, Other Fluids

- 22–25 °C Not recommended within 2 hours
- 2–8 °C   Not recommended within 2 hours
- –20 °C   Not recommended 2–4 weeks
  - **NOTE**: Do not freeze blood or bone marrow before lysing red blood cells (RBCs).
- –70 °C   Preferred storage condition
  - **NOTE**: Do not freeze blood or bone marrow before lysing red blood cells (RBCs)

Nucleic Acid Storage Requirements

Storage of DNA Specimens

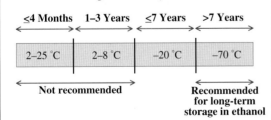

Nucleic Acid Preparation

Application?

DNA

- Amplification methods (PCR, LCR)
- Restriction enzyme digest
- Hybridization methods (Southern analysis)
- Sequencing

Nucleic Acid Preparation

Application?

RNA

- Amplification methods (RT-PCR)
- Hybridization methods (Northern analysis)

Nucleic Acid Preparation

Sample Source?

- Whole blood
- Buffy coat
- Serum or plasma
- Bone material
- Buccal cells
- Cultured cells

- Amniocytes or amniotic fluid
- Dried blood spots
- Fresh or frozen tissue (biopsy material)
- Sputum, urine, CSF, or other body fluids
- Fixed or paraffin-embedded tissue

Nucleic Acid Preparation

Other Considerations

What is the size or volume of each sample?
• Amount of DNA or RNA required
• Equipment and tube sizes required

How many samples are being processed?
• Capacity of the centrifuge
• Isolation method speed

Is a high-throughput or automated system available?
• 96-well plate methods
• Walk-away or semi-automation

Nucleic Acid Preparation

Choosing an Isolation Method

Important factors are:
• Processing speed
• Ease of use
• Yield of DNA or RNA
• Quality of DNA and RNA prepared
  (amplification performance)
• Shelf life/storage conditions
• Quality assurance criteria
• Cost of preparation

Basic Steps in Isolating DNA from Clinical Specimens

Separate WBCs from RBCs, if necessary
⬇
Lyse WBCs or other nucleated cells
⬇
Denature/digest proteins
⬇
Separate contaminants (*e.g.,* proteins, heme)
from DNA
⬇
Precipitate DNA if necessary
⬇
Resuspend DNA in final buffer

_____

_____

_____

_____

_____

_____

_____

_____

_____

_____

_____

_____

_____

_____

_____

_____

_____

_____

_____

DNA Isolation Methods
Liquid Phase Organic Extraction

- Phenol (50):chloroform/isoamyl alcohol (50:49:1)
- Lysed samples mixed with above; two layers are formed.
- Proteins remain at interface.
- DNA is removed with top aqueous layer.
- DNA is precipitated with alcohol and rehydrated.
- **Disadvantages**: slow, labor-intensive, toxic (phenol, chloroform), fume hood required, disposal of hazardous materials required

DNA Isolation Methods
Liquid Phase Nonorganic Salt Precipitation

- Cell membranes are lysed and proteins are denatured by detergent (such as SDS).
- RNA is removed with Rnase.
- Proteins are precipitated with salt solution.
- DNA is precipitated with alcohol and rehydrated.
- **Advantages**: fast and easy method, uses nontoxic materials, no fume hood required, no hazardous materials disposal issues, produces high-quality DNA

DNA Isolation Methods
Solid Phase Procedures

- Uses solid support columns, magnetic beads, or chelating agents
- Solid support columns: Fibrous or silica matrices bind DNA allowing separation from other contaminants.
- Magnetic beads: DNA binds to beads; beads are separated from other contaminants with magnet.
- Chelating resins
- **Advantages**: fast and easy, no precipitation required

DNA Purification Method Comparison

Liquid Phase	**Solid Phase**
(Lyse RBCs)	(Pre-lyse cells)
⬇	⬇
Lyse cells	Apply sample
⬇	⬇
(Protein digestion-ProK)	Wash
⬇	⬇
Separate proteins from DNA	Elute DNA
⬇	
Precipitate DNA-alcohol	
⬇	
Rehydrate DNA	

Basic Steps in Isolating RNA from Clinical Specimens

Separate WBCs from RBCs, if necessary

⬇

Lyse WBCs or other nucleated cells in presence
of protein denaturants, RNase inhibitors

⬇

Denature/digest proteins

⬇

Separate proteins, DNA, and contaminants
from RNA

⬇

Precipitate RNA if necessary

⬇

Resuspend RNA in final buffer

Precautions for Working with RNA in the Clinical Laboratory

RNA is not a stable molecule!
It is easily degraded by RNase enzymes.

- Use sterile, disposable plasticware (tubes, filter tips) marked "**For RNA Use Only**".
- Always wear gloves and work in a hood whenever possible/practical.
- Treat liquids with DEPC, except Tris-based buffers.

RNA Isolation Methods

Cesium Chloride Gradient

- Used mainly to get clean RNA for Northern blots
- Homogenize cells in guanidinium isothiocyanate and β-mercaptoethanol solution.
- Add to CsCl gradient and centrifuge for 12–20 hours; RNA will be at the bottom of tube.
- Re-dissolve in TE/SDS buffer.
- Precipitate RNA with salt and ethanol, then rehydrate.
- **Advantage**: high quality
- **Disadvantages**: extremely time-consuming, hazardous materials disposal issues

RNA Isolation Methods

Guanidinium-based Organic Isolation

- Phenol/guanidinium solution disrupts cells, solubilizes cell components, but maintains integrity of RNA.
- Add chloroform, mix, and centrifuge.
- Proteins/DNA remain at interface.
- RNA is removed with aqueous top layer.
- RNA is precipitated with alcohol and rehydrated.
- **Advantage**: faster than CsCl method
- **Disadvantages**: fume hood required, hazardous waste disposal issues

RNA Isolation Methods

Nonorganic Salt Precipitation

- Cell membranes are lysed and proteins are denatured by detergent (such as SDS) in the presence of EDTA or other RNase inhibitors.
- Proteins/DNA are precipitated with a high concentration salt solution.
- RNA is precipitated with alcohol and rehydrated.
- **Advantages:** fast and easy, nontoxic, produces high quality RNA

Resuspending Final Nucleic Acid Samples

Have some idea of expected nucleic acid yield.
Choose diluent volume according to
desired concentration.

Calculating Expected DNA Yield
Example: 1×10^7 cells $\times$ 6 pg DNA/cell $\times$ 80% yield
= 48 mg DNA

Resuspend DNA in TE buffer or ultrapure DNase-
free water. Resuspend RNA in ultrapure
RNase-free water.

Nucleic Acid Analysis

DNA or RNA is characterized using several
different methods for assessing quantity, quality,
and molecular size.

- UV spectrophotometry

- Agarose gel electrophoresis

- Fluorometry

- Colorimetric blotting

Components of a Spectrophotometer

- Stable source of radiant energy
  - UV, hydrogen lamp
  - Visible, tungsten filament lamp
- System of lenses and mirrors to focus the beam
- Monochromator (resolves radiation into
  wavelength bands)
- Transparent container for sample
- Detector
- Meter or recorder

Quantity from UV Spectrophotometry

- DNA and RNA absorb maximally at 260 nm.
- Proteins absorb at 280 nm.
- Background scatter absorbs at 320 nm.

Quantity from UV Spectrophotometry

[DNA] =

$(A_{260} - A_{320}) \times$ dilution factor $\times$ 50 µg/mL

[RNA] =

$(A_{260} - A_{320}) \times$ dilution factor $\times$ 40 µg/mL

Concentration = µg of DNA or RNA per mL of hydrating solution

---

Quantity from UV Spectrophotometry

Calculating Yield

Multiply the concentration of the DNA or RNA sample by the volume of hydrating solution added.

Example for DNA: 150 µg/mL $\times$ 0.1 mL = 15 µg

| Concentration from UV Spec. (µg DNA per ml of hydrating solution) | Volume of hydration solution | DNA yield |

Quality from UV Spectrophotometry

A_{260}/A_{280} = measure of purity

$(A_{260} - A_{320})/(A_{280} - A_{320})$

$1.7 - 2.0$ = good DNA or RNA

<1.7 = too much protein or
other contaminant (?)

Quality from Agarose Gel Electrophoresis

Genomic DNA: 0.6% to 1% gel, 0.125 µg/mL
ethidium bromide in gel and/or in running buffer

Electrophorese at 70–80 volts, 45–90 minutes.

Total RNA: 1% to 2% gel, 0.125 µg/ml ethidium
bromide in gel and/or in running buffer

Electrophorese at 80–100 volts, 20–40 minutes.

DNA Size from Agarose Gel Electrophoresis

Compares unknown DNA to known size standards

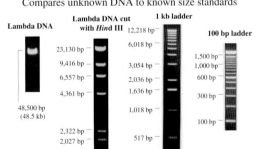

2/6/07

DNA Quality from Agarose Gel Electrophoresis

High molecular weight band (>48.5 kb)

Smearing indicates DNA degradation
(or too much DNA loaded).

DNA Quality from Agarose Gel Electrophoresis

Human Whole Blood DNA

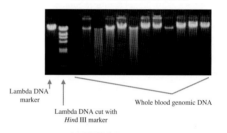

Lambda DNA
marker

Lambda DNA cut with
*Hin*d III marker

Whole blood genomic DNA

RNA Size and Quality from Agarose Gel Electrophoresis

Size: mRNA may be smaller or larger than ribosomal RNA (rRNA).

Quality: High-quality RNA has these characteristics:

- 28S rRNA band : 18S rRNA band = 2:1 intensity
- Little to no genomic DNA (high MW band)

Note: If 18S rRNA is more intense than 28S rRNA, or if both bands are smeared, RNA degradation is probable.

Cultured Cell RNA

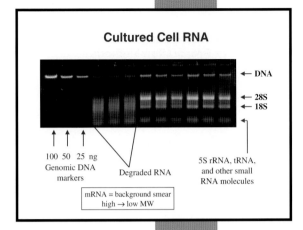

← DNA

← 28S
← 18S

100 50 25 ng
Genomic DNA
markers

Degraded RNA

5S rRNA, tRNA,
and other small
RNA molecules

mRNA = background smear
high → low MW

Storage Conditions

- Store DNA in TE buffer at 4 °C for weeks
  or at –20 °C to –80 °C for long term.

- Store RNA in Rnase-free ultrapure water at
  –70 °C.

Troubleshooting Nucleic Acid
Preparation Methods

Problem: No or low nucleic acid yield.

1. Make sure that ample time was allowed for
   resuspension or rehydration of sample.

   or

2. Repeat isolation from any remaining original
   sample (adjust procedure for possible low cell
   number or poorly handled starting material).

   or

3. Concentrate dilute nucleic acid using ethanol
   precipitation.

stop @ this slide
Go to section 7

_____

_____

_____

_____

_____

_____

_____

Troubleshooting Nucleic Acid Preparation Methods

Problem: Poor nucleic acid quality

1. If sample is degraded, repeat isolation from remaining original sample, if possible.

   or

2. If sample is contaminated with proteins or other substances, clean it up by re-isolating (improvement depends on the extraction procedure used).

DNA Replication and Repair

_____

_____

_____

_____

_____

_____

_____

_____

_____

_____

_____

_____

_____

_____

_____

_____

_____

_____

_____

Goal

To introduce basic concepts related to DNA replication and DNA repair, including the mechanism of eukaryotic DNA replication, DNA damaging agents, types of DNA damage, mechanisms of DNA repair, and genetic disorders related to faulty DNA repair.

Outline

- The eukaryotic cell cycle
- Origins of DNA replication
- Semiconservative DNA synthesis
- Types of DNA damage
- Mechanisms of DNA repair
- Genetic DNA repair deficiencies

Phases of the Cell Cycle

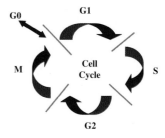

Eukaryotic DNA Replication

Eukaryotic chromosomes are composed of long linear DNA molecules that cannot be efficiently replicated in a continuous fashion. Therefore, replication of these large DNA molecules requires initiation of DNA replication from multiple sites (origins).

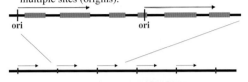

ori   ori

Origins of DNA Replication

Origins of replication are distributed throughout the genome, present every 50–100 kb. Not all origins are active at the same time during S phase.

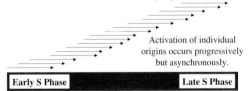

Activation of individual origins occurs progressively but asynchronously.

| Early S Phase | | Late S Phase |

S Phase (6–8 hours)

DNA Replication

DNA synthesis occurs bi-directionally from the origin, which in lower organisms consists of a **replicator** (cis-regulatory element) and an **initiator** (DNA binding protein complex).

41

_____

_____

_____

_____

_____

_____

_____

_____

_____

_____

_____

_____

_____

_____

_____

_____

_____

_____

_____

_____

Types of DNA Synthesis

- **DNA Replication:** Semi-conservative DNA synthesis associated with S phase of cell cycle in cell replication

- **Unscheduled DNA Synthesis:** DNA synthesis associated with DNA repair processes, occurring in all phases of cell cycle

Semiconservative DNA Synthesis

- Parental DNA strands act as templates for synthesis of new DNA, resulting in the synthesis of complementary daughter strands of newly synthesized DNA.

- In each newly generated cell, one strand of the DNA represents one of the parental strands of DNA, and the other is newly synthesized (semiconservative).

Semiconservative DNA Synthesis
(cont.)

- DNA is a unique biological molecule in that it carries all of the information required to perpetuate itself.

Semiconservative DNA Synthesis
Features of Eukaryotic DNA Replication

- Replication fork
- Leading strand
- Lagging strand (Okazaki fragments)
- DNA polymerase enzymes
- RNA primer (approximately 10 bases)

Semiconservative DNA Synthesis
The DNA Replication Fork

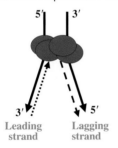

Semiconservative DNA Synthesis
Steps in DNA Replication

- Initiation

- Elongation

- Joining/Termination

Semiconservative DNA Synthesis
Initiation of DNA Replication

- Recognition of the origin (Ori) by a protein complex, termed the primosome.

- Separation of the parental DNA strands.

- Stabilization of the ssDNA regions.

- DNA synthesis begins at the replication fork.

Semiconservative DNA Synthesis
Elongation of DNA Strands

- Elongation requires a second protein complex, termed the replisome.

- Replisome moves along the DNA as it unwinds through the action of DNA helicase and gyrase enzymes.

- DNA daughter strands are synthesized by the DNA polymerase enzyme.

Eukaryotic DNA Polymerase Enzymes

- **Polymerase α**
  - Functions in nuclear replication and priming
- **Polymerase β**
  - Functions in nuclear DNA repair
- **Polymerase γ**
  - Functions in the replication of mitochondrial DNA
- **Polymerase δ**
  - Precise function unknown, possible nuclear polymerase

Semiconservative DNA Synthesis
Joining and Termination

- DNA strand joining at gaps between newly synthesized DNA strands is accomplished through the action of DNA ligase.

- The mechanism of replication termination is not currently known.

DNA Damage and Repair

DNA Damaging Agents

- Chemical and physical agents
  - X-rays
  - Ultraviolet light (UV)
  - Alkylating agents
  - Hydrogen ions
  - Other chemicals/mutagens
- Products of cellular metabolism

Types of DNA Damage

- Pyrimidine dimer
- Single- or double-strand breaks
- Base modifications
- Intercalation
- Base loss
- Interstrand cross-links

Types of DNA Damage

Pyrimidine Dimer

- Most often produced by UVC light.
- Represents the dimerization of thymine residues to form a cyclobutane ring.
- Less common are 6:4 photoproducts.

5′-AACCTTGCGTTCTAATTGCATGGCACA-3′

Types of DNA Damage

Single or Double Stranded Breaks

- Produced by a variety of DNA damaging agents.
- X-rays, fluorescent light, and others.
- Represents the scission of the phosphodiester bond on one or both DNA strands.

Single-strand break   Double-strand break

Types of DNA Damage

Base Modification
Produced by **Alkylation** of DNA

- Alkylating agents include methyl methane-sulfonate (MMS), N-methyl-N-nitrosurea (MNU).
- Most reactive sites in the DNA are the N^7 and O^6 positions of guanine, and the N^3 position of adenine.
- Alkylated bases mispair, producing mutation. Example: O^6-alkylguanine pairs with thymine rather than cytosine.

Types of DNA Damage

Base Modification

Other agents producing base modification of DNA:

- Polycyclic aromatic hydrocarbons—benzo(A)pyrene
- Aflatoxin B1—produced by mold on small grains (rice and peanuts); potent hepatocarcinogen
- Anthramycin—antitumor agent
- X-rays

Types of DNA Damage

DNA Intercalation

- Produced by the intercalation of drugs or other agents between adjacent base pairs in the DNA strand
- Causes distortion of the DNA double helix
- Intercalating agents include: Actinomycin D, Adriamycin, Daunomycin, and Ethidium Bromide

_____

_____

_____

_____

_____

_____

Types of DNA Damage

Interstrand Cross-links

- Product of covalent bonds formed between opposite strands of the DNA molecule
- Interstrand cross-links do not affect hydrogen bonding between DNA strands.
- Produced by exposure to nitrogen/sulfur mustards, platinum, mitomycin C, and psoralen + UV
- PUVA therapy for psoriasis = psoralen + UV

_____

_____

_____

_____

_____

_____

_____

Types of DNA Damage

Base Loss

- Represents depurination or depyrimidination of DNA
- Can result from various forms of DNA insult: Spontaneous chemical modification or modifications caused by various chemical agents

_____

_____

_____

_____

_____

_____

Types of DNA Damage

Base Loss *(cont.)*

- Results in the formation of **apurinic** or **apyrimidinic** sites
- Mechanism of base loss involves breakage of the glycosylic bond between the base and the deoxyribose moiety.

Mechanisms of DNA Repair

- Photoreactivation
- Direct rejoining
- Excision Repair (nucleotide excision repair, base excision repair)
- Methyltransferase
- Direct insertion
- Damaged DNA replication

DNA Repair Mechanisms
Photoreactivation

- Enzymes bind specifically to pyrimidine dimers that form at TT sites in the DNA in response to exposure to UVC.

- Enzyme catalyzes photolysis of cyclobutane ring linking the adjacent thymines.

- The enzyme separates from the repaired DNA following destruction of the cyclobutane ring.

DNA Repair Mechanisms
Direct Rejoining

- DNA repair mechanism that functions to repair single-stranded breaks in the DNA.

- Strands of DNA are directly rejoined through the action of polynucleotide ligase.

- The bases on either side of the break cannot be damaged for this form of repair to occur.

DNA Repair Mechanisms

Nucleotide Excision Repair

- Faulty bases are excised from the DNA strand.

- This form of repair attacks bulky DNA adducts and apurinic/apyrimidinic sites.

Mechanism
- Endonuclease enzyme detects the DNA lesion and makes a single-strand incision.
- Exonuclease enzyme excises the defective segment of DNA.
- DNA polymerase synthesizes new DNA to fill the gap.
- DNA ligase closes final gap.

DNA Repair Mechanisms

Base Excision Repair

- Targets alkylated and deaminated bases in the DNA.

- Repair is achieved through removal of the damaged base.

Mechanism
- DNA glycosylase catalyzes hydrolysis of glycosylic bond.
- AP endonuclease hydrolyzes phosphodiester bond.
- Exonuclease excises deoxyribose-phosphate residue.
- Polymerase and ligase enzymes fill gap in DNA strand.

DNA Repair Mechanisms

Base Excision Repair

Base excision repair for pyrimidine dimers involves a number of enzymatic activities:

- UV-specific endonuclease
- Pyrimidine dimer-specific DNA glycosylase
- Apyrimidinic (AP) endonuclease
- DNA polymerase
- DNA ligase

DNA Repair Mechanisms
Methyltransferase

- Methyltransferase enzyme functions in the repair of O^6-alkylguanine.

- Transfers a methyl group from guanine to itself, resulting in the inactivation of the enzyme.

- Different tissues express varying levels of this enzyme, producing different levels of protection from this form of DNA lesion.

DNA Repair Mechanisms
Direct Insertion

- Accomplished through the action of the purine insertase enzyme.

- Inserts purine into apurinic sites in the damaged DNA from available free purines.

DNA Repair Mechanisms
Damaged DNA Replication

- **Postreplication repair**—Replication machinery bypasses damaged areas; gaps containing damaged sites are subsequently repaired.

- **Continuous DNA synthesis**—Process generates no gaps as DNA damage is repaired during synthesis of new DNA. Consequently, this process is error-prone.

_____

_____

_____

_____

_____

_____

_____

_____

_____

_____

_____

_____

_____

_____

_____

_____

_____

_____

Pathologic Manifestations of Defective DNA Repair

- Mutagenesis

- Carcinogenesis

- Cell death

- Age-related decreases in DNA-repair proficiency result in increased susceptibility to DNA damage.

- Various genetic diseases

Human Diseases Related to DNA Repair Deficiency

- **Xeroderma pigmentosum** (XP): Patients are hypersensitive to UV light; patients often develop malignancies of the skin.

- **Ataxia telangiectasia** (AT): Patients are sensitive to gamma irradiation; patients develop neurological and skin lesions.

- **Fanconi's anemia:** Patients demonstrate aplastic anemia, growth retardation, and congenital anomalies; related to a deficiency in repair of DNA cross-links.

DNA Repair Genes

Excision Repair-associated Genes
- XPA, XPE (Photoproduct binding proteins)
- XPD, XPB, CSA, CSB (helicase enzymes, transcription-dependent)
- XPC
- ERCC gene family (nuclease enzymes)

Mismatch Repair-associated Genes
- hMLH1, hMSH2
- PMS1, PMS2
- GTBP

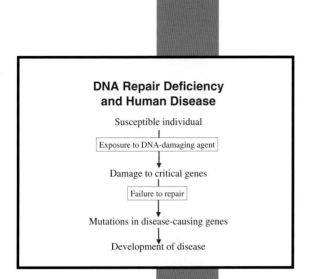

Gene Structure and Expression

_____

_____

_____

_____

_____

_____

_____

_____

_____

_____

_____

_____

_____

_____

_____

_____

_____

_____

Goal

To introduce basic concepts of gene structure, RNA transcription, RNA processing, regulation of gene expression, and protein synthesis.

Outline

- The central dogma of molecular biology
- Genes: Functional units of inheritance
- Gene structure
- RNA transcription
- RNA processing
- Translation

The Central Dogma of Molecular Biology

Defines the relationships between DNA, RNA, and protein in the transmission of genetic information into functional units of biological activity.

DNA $\longrightarrow$ RNA $\longrightarrow$ Protein

Functions of DNA

DNA serves two important functions contributing to cellular homeostasis:
1. Stable storage of genetic information
2. Transmission of genetic information

DNA provides the source of information for the synthesis of all the proteins in a cell, and it serves as a template for the faithful replication of genetic information that is ultimately passed into daughter cells.

Replication, Transcription, and Translation

Replication: the process of duplicating the genomic DNA through DNA-directed DNA synthesis.

Transcription: the process of generation of RNA from coding segments of DNA (genes).

Translation: the process of protein synthesis from the blueprint provided by the mRNA.

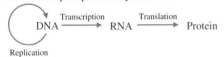

Genes
Functional Units of Inheritance

- Human genomic DNA contains several distinct types of sequences, including highly repetitive sequences, moderately repetitive sequences, and unique sequences.

- Highly repetitive sequences include Alu, LINE, and SINE sequences, whose precise functions are unknown.

Genes

Functional Units of Inheritance *(cont.)*

- Moderately repetitive sequences include genes for ribosomal RNAs (rRNAs) and transfer RNAs (tRNAs).

- Unique sequences typically correspond to structural genes, which encode for proteins, and many of which are single copy genes.

Structural Genes Encode Proteins

- The majority of structural genes in the human genome are much larger than necessary to encode their protein product.

- Structural genes are composed of coding and noncoding segments of DNA.

Structural Genes Encode Proteins

- The structure of a typical human gene includes informational sequences (coding segments termed exons) interrupted by noncoding segments of DNA (termed introns).

- The exon-intron–containing regions of genes are flanked by nontranscribed segments of DNA that contribute to gene regulation.

Gene Structure

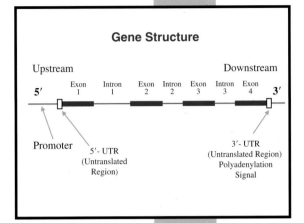

Upstream

Downstream

5′   Exon 1   Intron 1   Exon 2   Intron 2   Exon 3   Intron 3   Exon 4   3′

Promoter

5′- UTR
(Untranslated
Region)

3′- UTR
(Untranslated Region)
Polyadenylation
Signal

Control of Gene Expression

- Primary level of control is regulation of gene transcription activity.

- TATA box contained within the gene promoter provides binding sites for RNA polymerase.

- Enhancer sequences can be sited very far away from the gene promoter and provide for tissue-specific patterns of gene expression.

Gene Enhancer Sequences

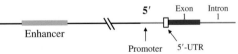

5′   Exon 1   Intron 1

Enhancer

Promoter   5′-UTR

1. Enhancer sequences are usually sited a long distance from the transcriptional start site.

2. Enhancers maintain a tissue-specific or cell-specific level of gene expression.

3. The gene promoter contains TATA box upstream of transcription start site.

_____

_____

_____

_____

_____

_____

_____

_____

_____

_____

_____

_____

_____

_____

_____

_____

_____

_____

_____

Transcription

- Transcription is the enzyme-dependent process of generating RNA from DNA.

- The process is catalyzed by a DNA-dependent RNA polymerase enzyme.

- Only "coding" segments of DNA (genes) are transcribed.

- Types of genes include structural genes (encode protein), transfer RNA (tRNA), and ribosomal RNA (rRNA).

Transcription

- Transition from DNA to RNA
- Initiation: Gene recognition
  - RNA polymerase enzyme and DNA form a stable complex at the gene promoter.
  - Promoter: Specific DNA sequence that acts as a transcription start site.
  - Synthesis of RNA proceeds using DNA as a template.
  - Only one strand (coding strand) is transcribed, the other strand has structural function.
  - Transcription factors are proteins that function in combination to recognize and regulate transcription of different genes.
- Termination signal

General Organization of a Eukaryotic Gene Promoter/Enhancer

Enhancer Region   Promoter Region

Regulatory Proteins   Regulatory Proteins   TFIID   RNA Polymerase II

TATA

200–2000 bp   100–200 bp   ~30 bp

200–10,000 bp

Transcription Factor Binding Sites in the Serum Albumin Gene

C/EBP HNF3 HNF3 NF1   NF1 C/EBP DBP NF-Y HNF1 TFIID

Enhancer Region   Promoter Region

RNA Polymerase Enzymes

(DNA-dependent RNA Polymerase)

- **RNA Polymerase I** transcribes most rRNA genes (RNA component of ribosomes).

- **RNA Polymerase II** transcribes structural genes that encode protein.

- **RNA Polymerase III** transcribes tRNA genes (for transfer RNAs).

- **RNA Polymerase IV** is the mitochondrial RNA polymerase enzyme.

Regulation of Gene Expression

- Specific regulatory sequences in the DNA located relative to the transcriptional start site are recognized and bound by specific proteins and protein complexes.

- These protein–DNA interactions can modify the level of gene transcription or the pattern of gene expression related to tissue or cell type.

_____

_____

_____

_____

_____

_____

_____

_____

_____

_____

_____

_____

_____

_____

_____

_____

_____

RNA Transcription and Processing

- The process of RNA transcription results in the generation of a primary RNA transcript (hnRNA) that contains both exons (coding segments) and introns (noncoding segments).

- The noncoding sequences must be removed from the primary RNA transcript during RNA processing to generate a mature mRNA transcript that can be properly translated into a protein product.

Nuclear Processing of RNA

- Chemical modification reactions (addition of the 5′ CAP)

- Splicing reactions (removal of intronic sequences)

- Polyadenylation (addition of the 3′ polyA tail)

RNA Processing

- Capping of the 5′-end of mRNA is required for efficient translation of the transcript (special nucleotide structure).

- Polyadenylation at the 3′-end of mRNA is thought to contribute to mRNA stability (PolyA tail).

- Once processed, the mature mRNA exits the nucleus and enters the cytoplasm where translation takes place.

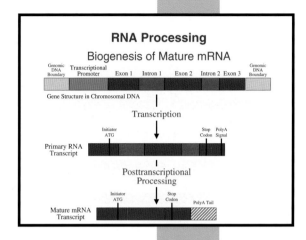

RNA Processing
Biogenesis of Mature mRNA

RNA Processing
Fundamentals of RNA Splicing

RNA Processing

- Ribonucleoproteins (snRNPs) function in RNA processing to remove intronic sequences from the primary RNA transcript (intron splicing).

- Alternative splicing allows for the generation of different mRNAs from the same primary RNA transcript by cutting and joining the RNA strand at different locations.

- snRNPs are composed of small RNA molecules and several protein molecules.

- Five subunits form the functional spliceosome.

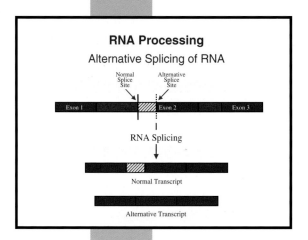

RNA Processing

Alternative Splicing of RNA

Normal Splice Site — Alternative Splice Site

Exon 1 | Exon 2 | Exon 3

RNA Splicing

Normal Transcript

Alternative Transcript

Translation

(Protein Synthesis)

- Translation occurs in the cytoplasm of the cell.

- It requires tRNA and rRNA species.

- tRNAs are recognized by aminoacyl tRNA synthetase enzymes, which attach amino acids to the 3′ attachment site of specific tRNA molecules.

- Each tRNA has a 3-base sequence (anticodon) that facilitates specific recognition and interaction with a codon in the mRNA.

The Universal Genetic Code

First Position (5′-end)	Second Position				Third Position (3′-end)
	U	C	A	G	
U	Phe	Ser	Tyr	Cys	U
U	Phe	Ser	Tyr	Cys	C
U	Leu	Ser	Stop	Stop	A
U	Leu	Ser	Stop	Trp	G
C	Leu	Pro	His	Arg	U
C	Leu	Pro	His	Arg	C
C	Leu	Pro	Gln	Arg	A
C	Leu	Pro	Gln	Arg	G
A	Ile	Thr	Asn	Ser	U
A	Ile	Thr	Asn	Ser	C
A	Ile	Thr	Lys	Arg	A
A	Met	Thr	Lys	Arg	G
G	Val	Ala	Asp	Gly	U
G	Val	Ala	Asp	Gly	C
G	Val	Ala	Glu	Gly	A
G	Val	Ala	Glu	Gly	G

Translation of mRNA

mRNA
5′…NNNNNNN**AUG**CUCGGGAGCCAU**UAA**NNNNN…3′

Translation Start Site

Translation Stop Signal

Codon Usage   AUG-CUC-GGG-AGC-CAU-UAA

Translation

Peptide Sequence   Met-Leu-Gly-Ser-His

SECTION

Mutation

_____

_____

_____

_____

_____

_____

_____

_____

_____

_____

_____

_____

_____

_____

_____

_____

_____

_____

_____

Goal

To introduce basic concepts related to mutation, including natural nucleotide sequence variations, types of mutations, mechanisms of mutation, and consequences of mutation.

Outline

- Basic concepts related to mutation
- Genetic polymorphisms
- RFLPs and VNTRs
- Types of mutations
- Frequency and origins of mutation
- Mechanisms of mutation
- Consequences of mutation

Molecular Diagnostics

The ability to discern useful information from molecular diagnostic assays is related to the development and application of molecular technologies that facilitate the direct visualization of nucleic acid sequence alterations, both those occurring naturally and those related to mutation.

Basic Concepts Related to Mutation

- Locus
- Allele
- Genetic polymorphism
- Mutation

Basic Concepts Related to Mutation
Genetic Locus

Locus refers to the position or location of a gene in the genome. Genetic loci are defined by chromosomal location, using chromosome bands (G-band or R-band) or molecular markers (microsatellites) as a point of reference.

Basic Concepts Related to Mutation
Allele

An allele is the "version" of a gene that is present at any given locus. Allelic differences are related to alterations in the nucleotide sequence of a gene.

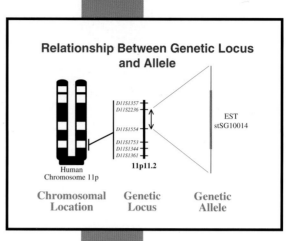

Relationship Between Genetic Locus and Allele

Human Chromosome 11p

11p11.2

EST stSG10014

Chromosomal Location **Genetic Locus** **Genetic Allele**

Basic Concepts Related to Mutation
Genetic Polymorphism

Polymorphism refers to the occurrence of multiple alleles at a locus, where at least two alleles appear with a frequency of >1% in the general population.

Genetic Polymorphisms

- Genetic polymorphisms are most often normal occurrences.
- Polymorphisms facilitate molecular tracking of clinically important genes.
- Identification of disease-related genes through positional mapping would be impossible without polymorphisms.
- There are numerous forms of variable DNA sequences.

Genetic Polymorphisms

- Every person has two copies of each chromosome (22 autosomes), except the sex chromosomes (XY). Therefore, every person has two copies of each gene ("unique" or "single-copy" genes).

- The DNA sequence of any particular polymorphism must be different at each allele to be "informative."

Genetic Polymorphism
Dinucleotide Microsatellite Repeat Polymorphism

Structural
Gene

Exon/
Intron Map

Intron 3

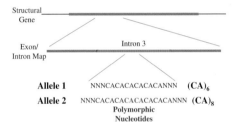

Allele 1	NNNCACACACACACANNN	$(CA)_6$
Allele 2	NNNCACACACACACACACANNN	$(CA)_8$

Polymorphic
Nucleotides

Genetic Polymorphism
Coding Sequence Polymorphism

Structural
Gene

Exon/
Intron Map

Exon 2

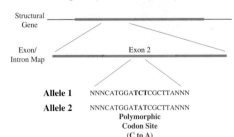

Allele 1	NNNCATGGA**TCT**CGCTTANNN
Allele 2	NNNCATGGA**TAT**CGCTTANNN

Polymorphic
Codon Site
(C to A)

Discrimination of Allelic Variation Using PCR

NNNCACACACACACANNN

NNNCACACACACACACACANNN

PCR

Electrophoretic Separation of Products
Amplicon 1 (200 bp)
Amplicon 2 (206 bp)

Genetic Polymorphism

Dinucleotide Microsatellite Repeat Polymorphism

Homozygous Individual (carries shorter alleles)   Heterozygous Individual (carries both alleles)   Homozygous Individual (carries longer alleles)

Polyacrylamide Gel

Discrimination of Genetic Polymorphisms by PCR

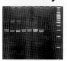 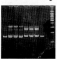

D15S822   *D3S1744*

Examples of polyacrylamide gel separation of PCR products from human tumor samples demonstrating informative allelic variations at two different genetic loci. Differences between tumor tissues and between individual patients can be seen.

Basic Concepts Related to Mutation
Gene Sequence Variation

- Nucleotide changes in a gene sequence can give rise to synthesis of an abnormal protein with altered structural and functional properties.
- Some nucleotide sequence changes do not alter the resulting protein product.
- Some nucleotide sequence changes are mutations, others are genetic polymorphisms.

Basic Concepts Related to Mutation
Polymorphisms and Mutations

- The majority of genetic polymorphisms do not represent mutations.

- Not all mutations are polymorphisms.

Basic Concepts Related to Mutation
Genetic Polymorphism

- Any two copies of human DNA will differ at 1/100 to 1/500 of all nucleotide positions.
- On average across the entire genome, 1/270 nucleotide positions will be polymorphic.
- **Human DNA is highly variable!**

Basic Concepts Related to Mutation

Types of Genetic Polymorphism

Certain types of polymorphism can be exploited in the development of molecular assays:

- **R**estriction **F**ragment **L**ength **P**olymorphisms (RFLPs)
- **V**ariable **N**umber of **T**andem **R**epeats (VNTR)

RFLPs and VNTRs are useful in molecular assays based upon the Southern blot.

Genetic Polymorphism

RFLP

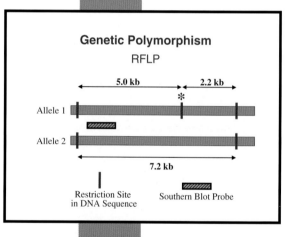

Genetic Polymorphism

RFLP

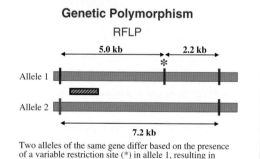

Two alleles of the same gene differ based on the presence of a variable restriction site (*) in allele 1, resulting in differing restriction patterns for these two gene segments. Placement of the probe (cross-hatch box) allows discernment of polymorphic alleles.

Genetic Polymorphism
RFLP

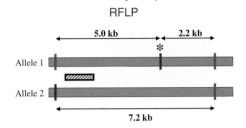

Restriction Digestion Results
- Allele 1: 5 kb and 2.2 kb DNA bands (variant bands)
- Allele 2: 7.2 kb DNA band (invariant band)

Genetic Polymorphism
RFLP

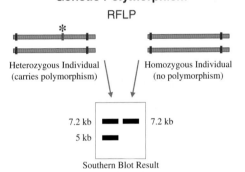

Genetic Polymorphism
VNTR

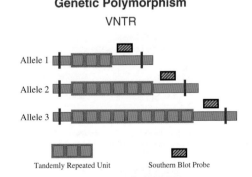

Genetic Polymorphism

VNTR

Alleles of the same gene differ based on the presence of a variable number of tandemly repeated units (red boxes), between invariant restriction sites, resulting in different sized restriction fragments from these gene segments.

Genetic Polymorphism

VNTR

Restriction Digest Results
- Allele 1 contains 3 repeat units, 200 bp restriction product.
- Allele 2 contains 6 repeat units, 230 bp restriction product.
- Allele 3 contains 9 repeat units, 260 bp restriction product.

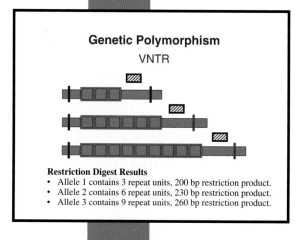

Genetic Polymorphism

VNTR

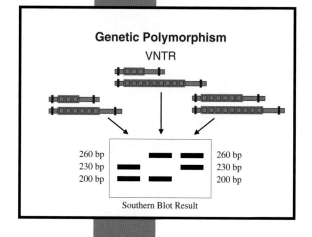

260 bp
230 bp
200 bp

260 bp
230 bp
200 bp

Southern Blot Result

Types of Genetic Lesions That Can Contribute to Disease Pathogenesis

- Aneuploidy (alteration of G1 DNA content)
- Chromosomal abnormalities (translocations, large deletions)
- Gene amplification (increase in gene copy number)
- Gene mutation (point mutation, insertional mutation, deletion)

Types of Genetic Lesions That Can Contribute to Disease Pathogenesis *cont.*

- Point mutation (alteration of individual nucleotides within a gene sequence)
- Insertional mutation (gain of a new sequence disrupting the coding sequence of a gene)
- Deletion (loss of gene segments)

Types of Mutations

Nucleotide Sequence Alterations
- Point mutations
- Insertions
- Deletions

Large-scale Alterations
- Chromosomal rearrangements
- Chromosomal deletion
- Gene amplification

Types of Mutations

Nucleotide Sequence Alterations

Point Mutations
- Transition/transversion
- Missense mutations (produces amino acid substitution in protein product)
- Nonsense mutation (produces premature STOP codon)
- Splice site mutation (intron/exon border, produces splice variant)

Types of Mutations

Nucleotide Sequence Alterations

Deletions and Insertions
- Frequently result in frameshift mutation related to the number of bases inserted or deleted from the DNA strand.
- A frameshift results from insertion or deletion of 1–2 bases, or 4–5 bases, or other numbers of bases that are not multiples of 3.
- Insertion or deletion of bases in multiples of 3 results in aberrant protein product containing new amino acids or lacking normal amino acid complement.

Chromosomal Alterations

Chromosomal Deletions
- Terminal deletion
- Interstitial deletion

Chromosomal Amplifications
- Amplification *in situ*
- Generation of double minute chromosomes

Chromosomal Rearrangements
- Chromosomal translocation
- Chromosomal inversion

Chromosomal Deletions

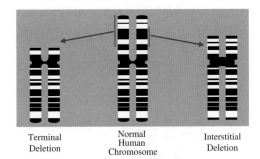

Terminal Deletion | Normal Human Chromosome | Interstitial Deletion

Chromosomal Amplification

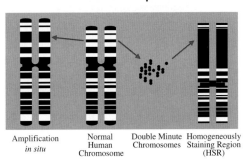

Amplification *in situ* | Normal Human Chromosome | Double Minute Chromosomes | Homogeneously Staining Region (HSR)

Chromosomal Rearrangements

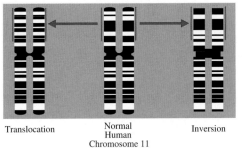

Translocation | Normal Human Chromosome 11 | Inversion

_____

_____

_____

_____

_____

_____

_____

_____

_____

_____

_____

_____

_____

_____

_____

_____

_____

_____

_____

_____

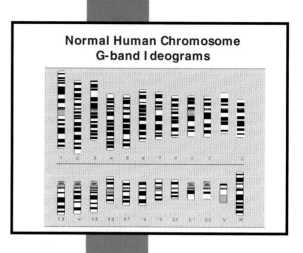

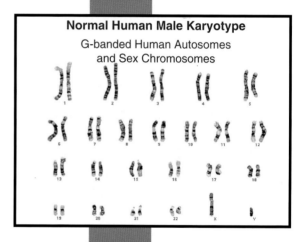

Gene Structure

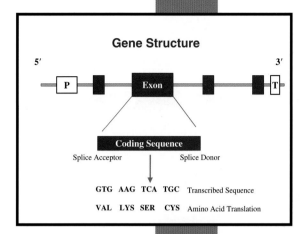

Types of Mutation
Missense Mutation

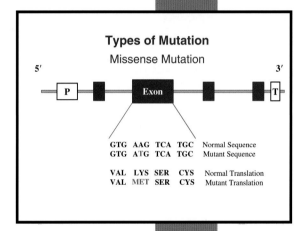

Activation of the c-H-*ras* Proto-oncogene by Point Mutation

Normal c-H-*ras*

1	2	3	4	5	6	7	8	9	10	11	12	13	188	189
Met	Thr	Glu	Tyr	Lys	Leu	Val	Val	Val	Gly	Ala	Gly	Gly	Leu	Ser

ATG ACG GAA TAT AAG CTG GTG GTG GTG GGC GCC GGC GGT ... CTC TCC

ATG ACG GAA TAT AAG CTG GTG GTG GTG GGC GCC GTC GGT ... CTC TCC

Met Thr Glu Tyr Lys Leu Val Val Val Gly Ala Val Gly Leu Ser

Mutant EJ-*ras*

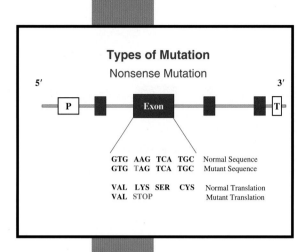

Types of Mutation

Nonsense Mutation

GTG	AAG	TCA	TGC	Normal Sequence
GTG	TAG	TCA	TGC	Mutant Sequence
VAL	LYS	SER	CYS	Normal Translation
VAL	STOP			Mutant Translation

Origin and Frequency of Mutations

Germline mutations occur in germ cells (eggs or sperm) and are passed from one generation to the next.

Somatic mutations occur in somatic cells, except mutations that are inherited through the germline.

1×10^{15} cell divisions occur in the lifetime of an organism, resulting in 1×10^{-10} replication errors (mutations).

What Contributes to the Mutation Rate in Normal Cells?

- Rates of DNA modification
- Rates of DNA chemical conversion
- Rates of DNA adduction
- Rates of DNA repair
- Cell cycle transit times

What is the Spontaneous Mutation Rate in Normal Cells?

Measured at the hypoxanthine-guanine phosphoribosyl-transferase (HPRT) locus:

Untransformed human cells (fibroblasts)
2.7×10^{-10} to 1×10^{-9}
mutations/nucleotide/cell generation

How Many Mutations Do Cells Accumulate During the Life of an Organism Due to Spontaneous Mutation?

At a rate of 1.4×10^{-10} mutations/nucleotide/cell generation, cells will accumulate approximately three mutations during the life of the organism.

Chemical Insult
N-nitroso Compounds
Polycyclic Aromatic Hydrocarbons
Crosslinking Agents

Spontaneous Chemical Modification

Physical Insult
Ionizing radiation
Ultraviolet Light

Genomic DNA

Damaged DNA
Bulky Adducts
Strand Breaks
Apurinic or Apyrimidinic Sites
Cyclobutane Pyrimidine Dimers
Crosslinks

Normal DNA Repair
Nucleotide Excision Repair
Enzymatic Reversal

Deficient DNA Repair
(with DNA replication)

Correction of Defect

Generation of Stable DNA Mutations

Factors Affecting Mutation in Normal Cells

- Slow repair of DNA damage—Genes located in regions of the genome that are subject to low levels of damage surveillance by repair enzymes are subject to increased mutation due to slow repair of damaged sites.

- Timing of gene replication—Genes replicated early in the S phase are subject to increased mutation frequency due to a lack of sufficient time for repair after damage and before replication of that portion of the genome.

Slow Repair of Damaged DNA

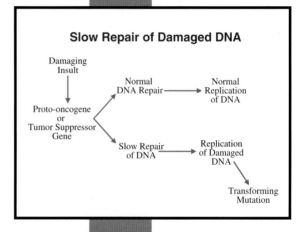

Timing of Replication and DNA Mutation

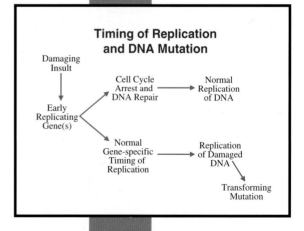

Timing of Replication of Cellular Proto-oncogenes and Tumor Suppressor Genes

Proto-oncogenes
c-abl, *c-erbA*, *c-erbB*, *c-fes*,
c-fms, *c-mos*, *c-myb*, *c-myc*,
c-neu, *c-ref*, *c-H-ras*, *c-K-ras*,
c-N-ras, *c-rel*, *c-sis*

Tumor Suppressor Genes
p53, Rb1

Proto-oncogenes
c-N-myc, *c-K-ras* (some cell lines)

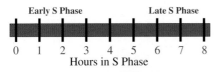

Early S Phase   **Late S Phase**

0   1   2   3   4   5   6   7   8
Hours in S Phase

Microsatellite Instability

- Mutations include repeat sequence *expansion* (representing insertional mutagenesis) or repeat sequence *contraction* (representing deletion mutagenesis).

- Mutations can affect mononucleotide repeats and/or higher order repeat sequences (dinucleotide, trinucleotide, tetranucleotide, etc.).

Microsatellite Instability in Human Tumors

N   T   N   T   N   T   N   T

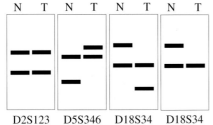

D2S123   D5S346   D18S34   D18S34
Normal   Expansion   Contraction   Deletion

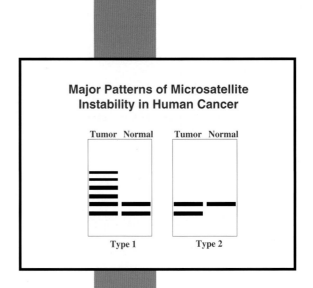

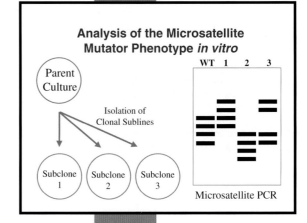

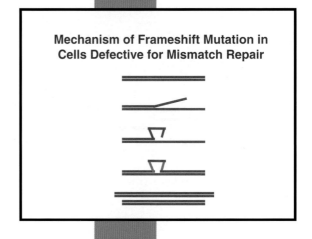

Mechanism of Frameshift Mutation in Cells Defective for Mismatch Repair

```
NNNCACACACACACANNN        Normal (CA)6
NNNGTGTGTGTGTGTNNN        Microsatellite Repeat
```
↓ DNA Replication

```
NNNCACACACA ⟶
NNNGTGTGTGTGTGTNNN
```
↓ Slippage on Template DNA Strand

```
NNNCACACA ⟶
NNNGTGTGTGTNNN
        GT
        TG    Formation of Stabilized Loop Domain
        GT
```
↓ Completion of Replication

↓ Second Round of Replication

```
NNNCACACACACACANNN        NNNCACACANNN
NNNGTGTGTGTGTGTNNN        NNNGTGTGTNNN
     Normal Allele        Contracted (Mutant) Allele
```

Mechanism of Frameshift Mutation in Cells Defective for Mismatch Repair

```
NNNCACACACACACANNN        Normal (CA)6
NNNGTGTGTGTGTGTNNN        Microsatellite Repeat
```
↓ DNA Replication

```
NNNCACACACA ⟶
NNNGTGTGTGTGTGTNNN
```
↓ Slippage on Replicating DNA Strand

```
        AC
        CA    Formation of Stabilized Loop Domain
        AC
NNNCACACACAC ⟶
NNNGTGTGTGTGTGTNNN
```
↓ Completion of Replication

↓ Second Round of Replication

```
NNNCACACACACACANNN        NNNCACACACACACACACANNN
NNNGTGTGTGTGTNNN          NNNGTGTGTGTGTGTGTGTNNN
     Normal Allele        Expanded (Mutant) Allele
```

What is the Microsatellite Mutation Rate in Normal Cells?

Measured using a selectable reporter system containing an artificial dinucleotide microsatellite repeat:

Untransformed Human Cells
(NHF1 Fibroblasts)
12.7×10^{-8} mutations/cell/generation

87

_____

_____

_____

_____

_____

_____

_____

Critical Targets of Microsatellite Mutation In Human Cancer

- *TGFβRII, IGFRII*—genes involved in suppression of cell proliferation

- *BAX*—genes involved in apoptosis

- *hMSH3, hMSH6*—mismatch repair genes

- *APC*—adenomatous polyposis coli tumor suppressor gene

Molecular Technologies

_____

_____

_____

_____

_____

_____

_____

_____

_____

_____

_____

_____

_____

_____

_____

_____

_____

_____

_____

_____

Goal

To introduce methods for preparing and analyzing nucleic acids, including standard laboratory techniques, methods for nucleic acid amplification and hybridization, and advanced methods for gene expression analysis.

Outline

- Diversity of genetic material
- Preparation of nucleic acids
- Basic techniques for analysis of nucleic acids
- Amplification methods and applications
- Hybridization methods and applications
- Microarray analysis of gene expression

Molecular Diagnostics

The tools (laboratory techniques) provided to us as a direct result of our understanding of molecular biology allow us to interrogate DNA/RNA for the purpose of identifying disease-causing genetic alterations.

Alleles and Loci

Allele refers to the "version" of a gene that is present at a given locus. Locus refers to a position or location of a gene on a chromosome.

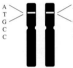
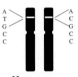

Two Copies of the Same Gene   Homozygous Alleles   Heterozygous Alleles

Diversity of Genetic Material

- Prokaryotic DNA

- Eukaryotic DNA

- Viral DNA or RNA

- Plasmid DNA

Prokaryotic DNA

- Genetic material is not compartmentalized into a nucleus.
- No complex protein: DNA structures (no histones).
- Prokayotes are haploid, containing one circular DNA molecule that carries a single copy of each gene.
- Prokaryotic DNA contains no intronic sequences.

Eukaryotic DNA

- Nuclear localization of genetic material.
- Multiple chromosomes, each representing a single linear DNA molecule.
- Complex protein:DNA interactions (histone proteins).
- Long noncoding DNA segments.

Viral Genetic Material

- Genetic information can be RNA or DNA.
- Both prokaryotes and eukaryotes serve as hosts.
- Nucleic acid is surrounded by a protein coat.
- Genetic material is either integrated into host genome or is replicated independently.

Plasmid DNA

- Plasmid DNA is a naked circular DNA molecule.
- Dependent on host cell for replication.
- Found most commonly in prokaryotes.

Isolating Nucleic Acids for Molecular Analysis

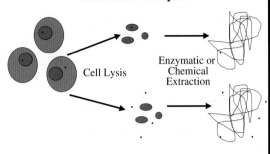

Cell Lysis

Enzymatic or Chemical Extraction

Preparation of Nucleic Acids
DNA Isolation

The purpose of DNA isolation/extraction procedures is to obtain useful samples of DNA that are free of contaminating molecules that will hinder DNA analysis.

Contaminating molecules include:

- **Cellular components** (such as protein)
- **Undesired reagents** (organics, salts, detergents)

Preparation of Nucleic Acids
DNA Isolation

Special considerations:

- **Degree of purity of DNA** (presence of contaminants)
- **Integrity of DNA**—High molecular weight versus low molecular weight(mechanical shearing and DNAse enzymes degrade DNA into smaller pieces)
- **Yield** (quantity of DNA prepared from a given amount of starting material)

- RNA is not stable & easily degradable

Preparation of Nucleic Acids
General DNA Isolation Procedure

Harvest Nucleated Cells

↓

Lyse Cells
- Detergent dissolves cell membrane and denatures protein.
- EDTA chelates divalent cations required by nucleases.
- Proteinase K degrades proteins.

Organic Extraction
- Uses phenol:chloroform:isoamyl alcohol
- Dissolves hydrophobic contaminants
- Denatures and removes proteins
- Aqueous phase:Organic phase
- DNA precipitation

Nonorganic Extraction
- Protein precipitation
- DNA precipitation

Preparation of Nucleic Acids
RNA Isolation

General considerations
- RNA is easily degraded by RNAse enzymes.
- Tissue culture serum contains high levels of RNAse. Certain tissues contain high levels of RNAse (placenta, liver, some tumors).
- Ribonucleases (RNAse) are very hardy enzymes. Inactivation requires 2 hours at 200 °C or 30 minutes in 1 M NaOH.
- Guanidinium isothiocyanate is a denaturing agent that inactivates RNAse.

Preparation of Nucleic Acids
Determination of Nucleic Acid Yield and Purity

- Spectrophotometry
  - Absorbance at 260 nm and 280 nm
  - 260 nm: concentration of DNA in sample
    - **OD = 1, 50 µg/mL dsDNA; 40 µg/mL ssDNA or RNA**
  - 260:280 ratio estimates purity
    - **1.8–2.0 = high purity**
    - **<1.8 = contamination with protein or phenol**
- EtBr fluorescence (gel electrophoresis)

Calculation of DNA Concentration

1. Start with 3 mL whole blood
2. Remove 300 µL for extraction
3. Reconstitute DNA in 100 µL buffer
4. $OD_{260} = 1.0$

$$1.0 \times 50\ \mu g/mL = 50\ \mu g/mL \times 100\ \mu L \times 1\ mL/1000\ \mu L = 5\ \mu g/\mu L$$

You now have 5 µg/µL in DNA buffer from the 300 µL blood.
If you extracted the entire 3 mL of blood from this patient,
what would your final concentration be?

Answer: 50 µg/µL if reconstituted in 100 µL buffer

Calculation of DNA Concentration

5 µL of reconstituted DNA is added to 995 µL water
for absorbance spectrophotometry.

Dilution factor
(5 µL in 995 µL)

$$\frac{A260 \times 50\ \mu g/mL \times 200}{1000\ \mu L/mL} = \mu g/\mu L\ DNA$$

Total volume of dilution

Basic Techniques for Analysis of Nucleic Acids

- Enzymatic modification (polymerase, kinase, phophatase, ligase)

- Endonuclease digestion (DNAse, RNAse, restriction enzymes) — *cut DNA up* — *have spec. cut sites*

- Electrophoresis (agarose and polyacrylamide gel electrophoresis)

95

cut sugar phosphate

Nucleic Acid Modifying Enzymes

- Restriction endonucleases ("molecular scapels")

- DNA polymerases (synthesize DNA)

- DNA ligases (join DNA strands by forming a phosphodiester bond)

- Kinases (phosphorylation of 5′-terminus of DNA molecule)

Nucleic Acid Modifying Enzymes
(cont.)

- Phosphatases (dephosphorylate 5′-terminus of DNA molecule)

- Ribonucleases (digest RNA molecule. Example: RNAse A)

- Deoxyribonucleases (digest DNA molecules)

---

we actually use only about 400

Nucleic Acid Modifying Enzymes
Restriction Endonucleases

- Found only in microorganisms
- Exhibit novel DNA sequence specificities
- >2000 distinct restriction enzymes have been identified
- Function as homodimers; recognize symmetrical dsDNA
- Utilized in the digestion of DNA molecules for hybridization procedures (Southern blot) or in the direct identification of mutations

Nucleic Acid Modifying Enzymes
Restriction Endonucleases *(cont.)*

- Recognize specific sequences of 4, 5, or 6 nucleotides
- Cut by breaking the phosphodiester bond in both strands
- Cutting genomic DNA with a RE results in many fragments of different sizes
- The smaller the recognition sequence the larger the number of fragments produced

Handwritten notes:
- verry specific
- can recog. 4-10 bp
- every 256 bp - should run into a cut site
- break sugar phosphate backbone

Restriction Enzymes

Cohesive Ends (5′ Overhang)	Cohesive Ends (3′ Overhang)	Blunt Ends (No Overhang)
BamH1	KpnI	HaeIII
GGATCC CCTAGG	GGTACC CCATGG	GGCC CCGG

Restriction Enzymes

GGATCC CCTAGG	AGATCT TCTAGA	CTCGTG GAGCAG	NNCAGTGNN NNGTCACNN
*Bam*HI (5′ Overhang)	*Bgl*II (5′ Overhang)	*Bss*SI (5′ Overhang)	*Tsp*RI (3′ Overhang)
Enzymes Generating Compatible Cohesive Ends		Enzymes Recognizing Nonpalindromic Sequences	

GATC CTAG	GGCC CCGG	CCCGGG GGGCCC	CCCGGG GGGCCC
*Dpn*I (Requires methylation)	*Hae*III (Inhibited by methylation)	*Sma*I (Blunt Ends)	*Xma*I (5′ Overhang)
Methylation-sensitive Enzymes		Isoschizomers	

97

_____

_____

_____

_____

_____

_____

Nucleic Acid Modifying Enzymes

Restriction Digestion of DNA

Restriction enzyme activity is measured in units (U)
Use 10 U of enzyme activity per µg of DNA.

To digest 10 µg DNA (concentration = 0.5 µg/µL) with
a restriction enzyme (RE) at concentration of (50 U/µL),
how much <u>DNA</u> do you need?

0.5 µg/µL = 10 µg/X

10 µg × (µL/0.5 µg) = X

X = 20 µL

_____

_____

_____

_____

_____

_____

_____

Nucleic Acid Modifying Enzymes

Restriction Digestion of DNA

To digest 10 µg DNA (concentration = 0.5 µg/µL)
with a RE at concentration of (50 U/µL),
how much <u>restriction enzyme</u> do you need?

10 µg × (10 U enzyme/µg DNA) × (1 µL/50 U enzyme) = 2 µL

The reaction also contains a buffer that is specific for
the restriction enzyme being used (NaCl concentration
is most important).

Buffers are added from a 10X stock. Distilled water
is used for the balance of reaction volume.

NOTE: The volume of enzyme should not be greater
than 10% of the total reaction volume.

_____

_____

_____

_____

_____

_____

_____

Nucleic Acid Modifying Enzymes

Typical Restriction Digestion Reaction

Reactions are composed of DNA template,
restriction enzyme, 10X buffer, and distilled
water. The required amounts of these components
can be calculated based on the number of
specimens to be digested:

- µL DNA
- µL restriction enzyme
- µL 10X buffer
- µL distilled water

Electrophoresis of Nucleic Acids

- Nucleic acids are separated based on size and charge.

- DNA molecules migrate in an electrical field at a rate that is inversely proportional to the $\log_{10}$ of molecular size (number of base pairs).

- Employs a sieve-like matrix (agarose or polyacrylamide) and an electrical field.

- DNA possesses a net negative charge and migrates towards the positively charged anode.

Applications of Electrophoretic Techniques in the Molecular Diagnostics Laboratory

Sizing of Nucleic Acid Molecules
- DNA fragments for Southern transfer analysis
- RNA molecules for Northern transfer analysis
- Analytical separation of PCR products

Detection of Mutations or Sequence Variations
- Single-strand conformational polymorphism (SSCP)
- Heteroduplex analysis (HA)
- Others (DGGE, etc.)

Electrophoresis of Nucleic Acids

Polyacrylamide Gel Electrophoresis (PAGE)

Advantages
- High degree of resolving power.
- Can effectively and reproducibly separate molecules displaying 1 bp differences in molecular size.
- Optimal separation is achieved with nucleic acids that are 5–500 bp in size.

gels run vertical

— limited can't go above or below

99

Electrophoresis of Nucleic Acids

Polyacrylamide Gel Electrophoresis
(PAGE) *(cont.)*

Typical Conditions

• Vertical gel setup, TBE buffer
(Tris-borate/EDTA) and constant power.

Disadvantages

• Acrylamide monomer is a neurotoxin.

• Polyacrylamide gels can be difficult to handle.

Polyacrylamide Gel Electrophoresis

Vertical Gel Format

Reservoir/Tank
Power Supply
Glass Plates, Spacers, and Combs

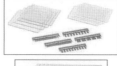

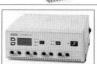

www.biorad.com

Electrophoresis of Nucleic Acids

Agarose Gel Electrophoresis

Advantages

• Greater range of separation of nucleic acid
molecules.

• Optimal separation is achieved with nucleic
acids that are 200 bp to 30 kb in size.

• Ease of preparation and handling.

Electrophoresis of Nucleic Acids

Agarose Gel Electrophoresis *(cont.)*

Typical Conditions

- Horizontal gel setup, TAE (Tris-acetate/EDTA) or TBE buffer and constant voltage.

Disadvantages

- Lower resolving power than PAGE.

Agarose Gel Electrophoresis

Horizontal Gel Format

Reservoir/Tank
Power Supply
Casting Tray and Combs

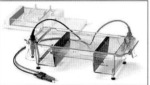 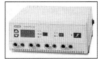

www.biorad.com

Electrophoresis of Nucleic Acids

TAE Buffer

- Composed of tris-acetate and EDTA (Tris base, pH adjusted with acetic acid)

- Useful in procedures where recovery of DNA is desired; used in electrophoresis of large DNA fragments

- Low buffering capacity; requires recirculation of buffer for some applications

- Increases migration of DNA through the gel

_____

_____

_____

_____

_____

_____

_____

_____

_____

_____

_____

_____

_____

_____

_____

_____

_____

_____

Electrophoresis of Nucleic Acids
TBE Buffer

- Composed of Tris-borate and EDTA (Tris base, pH adjusted with boric acid)
- Used in electrophoresis of smaller DNA fragments; produces better resolution of small DNA fragments
- High buffering capacity due to high ionic strength; does not require recirculation of buffer
- Decreases migration of DNA through the gel

Electrophoresis of Nucleic Acids
Preparation of DNA for Electrophoresis

- Add an appropriate loading buffer to the DNA sample (loading buffer contains glycerol, buffer, and one or more tracking dyes, such as bromophenol blue).
- Load DNA sample into the appropriate well of the gel.
- Document and verify loading order of the samples.
- Take care to minimize spillover or carryover into adjacent wells.

Electrophoresis of Nucleic Acids
Selection of Aragose Gel

Different concentrations of agarose in the gel solution affect the resolution and separation power of the gel.

- Use 4–6% agarose for separations of DNA molecules with small size variations.
- Use 0.5–1% for separation of restriction digested DNA fragments for Southern transfer analysis.

Example: Use 4% agarose to resolve a 3 bp difference in DNA fragment size.

Electrophoresis of Nucleic Acids
Preparation of Aragose Gel

- Choose an appropriate buffering system (TAE or TBE).
- Select a proper comb for formation of sample wells.
- Dissolve agarose in buffer solution by micro-waving.
- Allow gel solution to cool, pour, and polymerize.

Electrophoresis of Nucleic Acids
Preparation of Aragose Gel *(cont.)*

- Prepare DNA samples by adding loading buffer.
- Document and verify loading order of samples.
- Document electrophoretic conditions (voltage).
- Stain gel, visualize DNA, photograph/document.
- Dispose of gel properly.

Agarose Electrophoresis of Restriction Enzyme Digested Genomic DNA

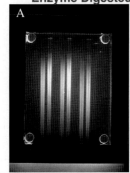 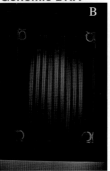

Electrophoresis of Nucleic Acids

Selection of Polyacrylamide Gel

Different concentrations of polyacrylamide in the gel affect the resolution and separation power of the gel.

- Use 10–15% polyacrylamide for separation of short oligonucleotides.

- Use 5–8% for DNA sequencing reactions.

Electrophoresis of Nucleic Acids

Selection of Polyacrylamide Gel *(cont.)*

Polyacrylamide Gel Variations
- Denaturing polyacrylamide gel electrophoresis (Mutation Detection Electrophoresis, MDE)
- Nondenaturing polyacrylamide gel electrophoresis (Single Strand Conformational Polymorphism, SSCP)

Electrophoresis of Nucleic Acids

Preparation of Polyacrylamide Gel

- Prepare an appropriate acrylamide solution (%). Denaturing gels (containing urea or other denaturant) are used when samples are denatured, "native" (nondenaturing) gels are used for native DNA.

- Add ammonium persulfate and TEMED to catalyze polymerization reaction.

Electrophoresis of Nucleic Acids
Preparation of Polyacrylamide Gel *(cont.)*

- Pour into glass plate gel sandwich and polymerize.
- Prepare DNA samples by adding loading buffer.
- Document and verify loading order of samples and electrophoretic conditions (voltage).
- Stain gel, visualize DNA, photograph/document and dispose of gel properly.

Polyacrylamide Gel Resolution of a Single PCR Product

Lane 1, blank; lane 2, negative; lane 3 positive; lane 4 and 5, polyclonal; lane 6 and 7, clonal band

Polyacrylamide Gel Electrophoresis of Restriction Digested PCR Products

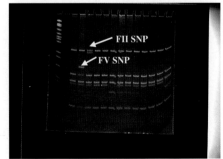

Quality Assurance Issues

- Document loading order of gel.
- Always include molecular size standards.
- Document electrophoresis conditions (matrix batch, apparatus employed, volt-hours run, etc.).
- Document results appropriately (photography, autoradiology, chemilumigram).

Factors Affecting Migration Rate

- Matrix type and porosity (%)
- Net charge of nucleic acid molecule
- DNA conformation
- Electric field strength
- Temperature of gel
- Nucleic acid base composition
- Presence of intercalating dyes
- Type and strength of buffer

Pulsed Field Gel Electrophoresis of DNA (PFGE)

PFGE is employed in the analysis of DNA fragments that are up to 100 kb in size. Separation is accomplished using a pulsed electrical field. PFGE is commonly used for genotyping prokaryotes.

PFGE of Bacterial DNA

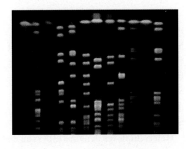

Single-stranded Conformational Polymorphism Analysis (SSCP)

- Mutation screening technique
- Short PCR products (<300 bp)
- Radiolabeled amplicons can be used for detection when small amounts of DNA are analyzed.
- Denature PCR amplicons using heat nondenaturing gel electrophoresis.
- Single-stranded DNA adopts a three-dimensional shape upon cooling.

Variations in mobility indicative of mutations reflect differences in conformation.

2/13/07

SSCP Analysis of PCR Products

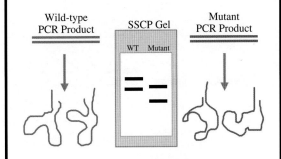

- Mix samples, ↑ temp to
denature & slowly cool to Rt
- Migration slower if DNA
mis-match occurs

Detection - DNA is not visible to eye
stain DNA w/ intercalating agents
bright strand
works @ low [ ]
- ethidium bromide = mutagen
- silver stain - heavy metal (toxicity d
poisoning)
- SYBR green - less mutagenic than
ethidium bromide
↑ conc. than etbr
5x

AT
&
CG → emit

Go to page 149

Heteroduplex Analysis (HA)

- Mutation screening technique
- PCR amplify DNA region of interest
- Mix patient (possible mutant) and control DNA samples
- Denature PCR amplicons using heat
- Slowly cool to room temperature
- Add denaturing loading buffer
- Electrophoresis using MDE gel matrix

Heteroduplexes demonstrate retarded migration due to sequence mismatches.

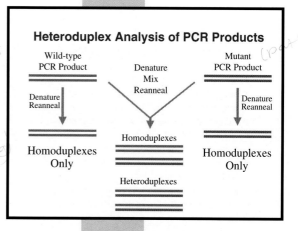

Heteroduplex Analysis of PCR Products

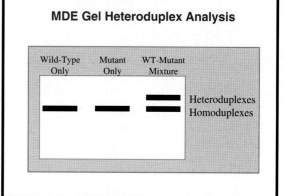

MDE Gel Heteroduplex Analysis

Capillary Zone Electrophoresis (CZE)

- Fragment size and sequence analysis
- Electrophoresis through capillary-containing polyacrylamide
- Detection of fluorescently labeled amplicons
- Internal size standards for computation of fragment sizes

Gel Electrophoresis
Troubleshooting

Arrested Migration of Nucleic Acid
- Buffer leak?
- Depletion of electrolytes?
- Power supply problem?

Abnormal Migration of Nucleic Acid
- Bubbles in gel?
- Overloaded samples?
- Loading buffer irregularities?
- Electrophoresis buffer irregularity?

Principles of Electrophoresis
Stoke's Law

- The forces that drive the analyte through the gel are the net charge of the molecule and the electric field strength.
- The forces that retard the movement of the molecule are the frictional forces, the pore size of the matrix, and size and shape of the molecule.
- The opposition of the acceleration of the analyte by the frictional forces is described by Stoke's Law.

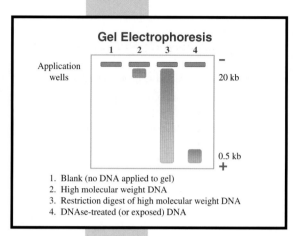

Gel Electrophoresis

Application wells

20 kb

0.5 kb

1. Blank (no DNA applied to gel)
2. High molecular weight DNA
3. Restriction digest of high molecular weight DNA
4. DNAse-treated (or exposed) DNA

2/20/07

Amplification of Nucleic Acids *in vitro*

Approaches to Amplification

Amplification of copy number—Includes enzyme-mediated amplification techniques that result in the synthesis of new copies of target sequences in the template DNA.

Amplification of signal—Includes techniques that increase detection sensitivity by amplification of detection signals rather than by increasing the copy number of the target sequence.

Amplification of Nucleic Acids *in vitro*

Amplification of Copy Number

- Polymerase chain reaction (PCR)

- Ligase chain reaction (LCR)

- Nucleic acid sequence-based amplification (NASBA)

- Transcription-mediated amplification (TMA)

- Strand-displacement amplification (SDA)

Amplification of Nucleic Acids *in vitro*
Signal Amplification

- Branched DNA (bDNA)

- Hybrid capture assay (HCA)

Amplification Techniques
Polymerase Chain Reaction

The polymerase chain reaction is a technique for the *in vitro* amplification of specific DNA sequences by primer extension of complementary strands of DNA.

The Polymerase Chain Reaction

A basic method for amplification of small target sequences from DNA (or RNA) that uses a thermostable DNA polymerase (such as *Taq* polymerase)

- Amplified DNA can be directly cloned or sequenced.

- Amplified DNA products are employed in various analytical electrophoretic techniques.

- Amplified DNA products can serve as probes in northern or Southern blot analyses.

The Polymerase Chain Reaction

- Solution-phase PCR (standard)
- RT-PCR (reverse transcription)
- *In situ* PCR (amplification on tissue section)
- PSM (PCR-mediated site-directed mutagenesis)
- RAPID (random amplified polymoprphic DNA)
- RCPCR (recombinant circle PCR)
- ASPCR (allele-specific PCR)

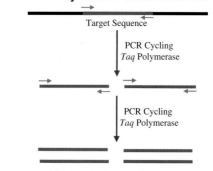

The Polymerase Chain Reaction

Target Sequence

PCR Cycling
Taq Polymerase

PCR Cycling
Taq Polymerase

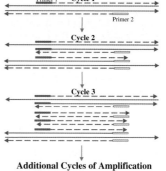

The Polymerase Chain Reaction

Primer 1 — **Cycle 1**

Primer 2

Cycle 2

Cycle 3

Additional Cycles of Amplification

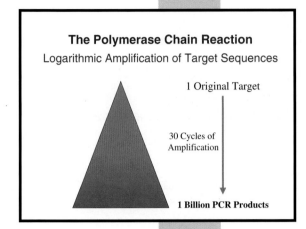

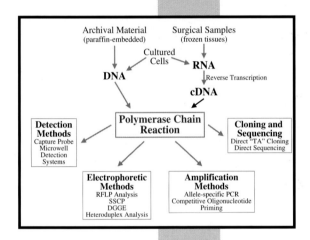

✱ Major slide

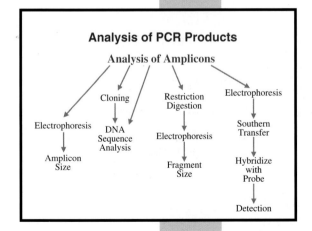

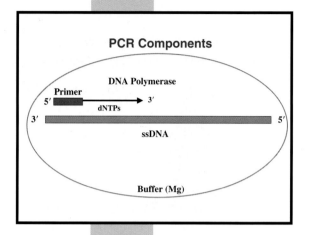

PCR Components

- DNA polymerase (Taq)(0.5–2 units): Heat stable

- Deoxynucleoside triphosphates (dNTPs) (200 uM)

- Reaction buffer: 10 mM TRIS (pH 8.4), 50 mM KCl, 1.5 mM MgCl$_2$, 0.001%gelatin

- Primers or oligonucleotides (15–25 bp): GC content (45–60%)

- Target DNA (ssDNA)

Troubleshooting PCR

- Too much of any of the PCR components can lead to nonspecific amplification (mispriming, thermodynamic infidelity).

- Too little of any of the PCR components can lead to no amplification.

The PCR Cycle

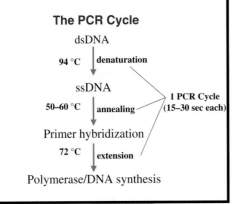

dsDNA

94 °C ↓ denaturation

ssDNA

50–60 °C ↓ annealing

Primer hybridization

72 °C ↓ extension

Polymerase/DNA synthesis

1 PCR Cycle
(15–30 sec each)

Polymerase Chain Reaction

Standard PCR Reaction

25–100 ng DNA template
50 mM KCl
10 mM Tris HCl (pH 8.4)
1.5 mM $MgCl_2$
gelatin
0.25 mmoles each primer
200 µM each dNTP
2.5 U *Taq* polymerase

***In Vitro* Amplification**

How much amplification do you get?

Amplicons = A 2^{n-2}

n = number of cycles

A = starting target copy number

Reagent limitations and polymerase infidelity
result in plateau effect
(reduced amplification efficiency).

_____

_____

_____

_____

_____

_____

_____

Polymerase Chain Reaction

Controls for PCR

- Blank reaction
  - Controls for contamination
  - Contains all reagents except DNA template

- Negative control reaction
  - Controls for specificity of the amplification reaction
  - Contains all reagents and a DNA template lacking the target sequence

---

_____

_____

_____

_____

_____

_____

_____

Polymerase Chain Reaction

Controls for PCR *(cont.)*

- Positive control reaction

  - Controls for sensitivity

  - Contains all reagents and a known target-containing DNA template

---

_____

_____

_____

_____

_____

_____

_____

Effect of MgCl$_2$ Concentration on PCR Amplification

Molecular Marker   Increasing [Mg^{++}]

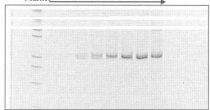

0.5 0.75 1.0 1.25 1.5 2.0 3.0 4.0

Mg^{++} Concentration (mM)

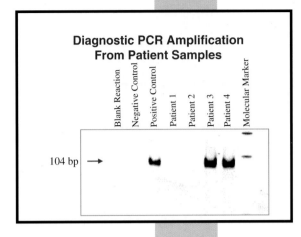

**Diagnostic PCR Amplification
From Patient Samples**

104 bp →

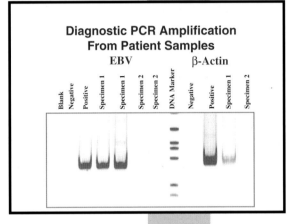

**Diagnostic PCR Amplification
From Patient Samples**

EBV   β-Actin

Advantages of PCR

• PCR is fast (2–5 hours).

• DNA or RNA can be amplified.

• High-yield amplification can be achieved (10^6 to 10^9 amplification).

_____

_____

_____

_____

_____

_____

_____

_____

_____

_____

_____

_____

_____

_____

_____

_____

_____

_____

Advantages of PCR _(cont.)_

- DNA from one cell equivalent can be amplified.

- PCR products can be directly sequenced.

- PCR products can be directly cloned.

- DNA sequences up to 30 kb can be amplified.

Disadvantages of PCR

- Must know the sequence of the DNA of interest.
- Highly susceptible to contamination or false amplification.
- Amplification may not be 100% specific.
- Specificity of amplification is dependent on temperature and Mg^{++} concentration.
- Analysis and product detection usually takes longer than the PCR reaction itself.

Troubleshooting PCR

- No PCR product
  - Verify that all components were added to the reaction.
  - Check pipettors and reagents.
  - Check detection method.
- Too many bands
  - Specificity of primers.
  - Annealing temp too low, excessive Mg^{++} or cycles.

Troubleshooting PCR *(cont.)*

- Primer dimers
  - Size is the sum of two primer lengths.
  - Taq extends one primer, which is annealed to another primer.
  - Annealing temperature too low, excess primers.

PCR Inhibitors

- Detergent
- Phenol
- Heparin
- Heme
- Dyes (bromphenol blue)
- CSF, urine, sputum, paraffin

  ***Dilute extracted DNA.**

Contamination of PCR Reactions

- Most common cause is carelessness and bad technique.
- Separate pre- and post-PCR facilities.
- Dedicated pipettors and reagents.
- Change gloves.
- Aerosol barrier pipette tips.
- ***Meticulous technique

  | 10% bleach, acid baths, UV light |

Uracil-N-Glycosylase (UNG)

1. Substitute dUTP for dTTP in initial PCR mix.

2. Proceed with PCR and detection.

3. In the next PCR to be set up, initial 30 min incubation at 37 °C.

4. UNG will destroy any dUTP containing DNA products.

In Vitro **Amplification**

Signal Amplification

Sensitivity of detection of product is dependent on amplification of signal, rather than amplification of the product itself.

- Branched DNA (bDNA)
- Hybrid capture assay (HCA)

Reverse Transcription

Reverse transcription is the process through which a single-stranded RNA molecule gives rise to a complementary DNA (cDNA) molecule through a primer-dependent polymerase-dependent reaction.

"First Strand Synthesis"

Reverse Transcription-Polymerase Chain Reaction (RT-PCR)

Steps in the RT-PCR reaction:

- RNA isolation
- Reverse transcription
- PCR amplification
- Analysis of PCR product

Reverse Transcription of RNA (RT)

Primer Options for RT reaction
- Oligo(dT)
- Random Hexamers
- Sequence-specific Primers

Enzyme Options for RT Reaction
- Retroviral RNA-directed DNA polymerase
- AMV Reverse Transcriptase (avian myeloblastosis virus)
- MMLV Reverse Transcriptase (moloney murine leukemia virus)

The Polymerase Chain Reaction

Amplification Methods for Mutation Detection

- Allele-specific amplification (uses sequence-specific primers for wild-type and mutant alleles)

- Competitive oligonucleotide priming (uses sequence-specific primers for wild-type and mutant alleles that are present in the same reaction mixture)

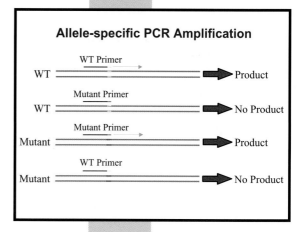

Allele-specific PCR Amplification

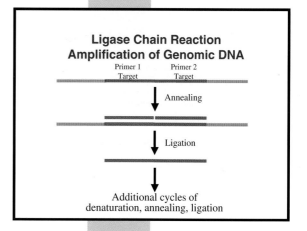

Ligase Chain Reaction Amplification of Genomic DNA

- Two primers are directed against adjacent target sequences.
- Successfully annealed primers are ligated together through the action of a thermostable DNA ligase (amplification is accomplished through successive cycles of annealing and ligation).
- Useful for detection of specific mutations in gene sequences.
- Adapted for diagnostic testing of some infectious agents (chlamydia, gonorrhea, listeria, and HPV).

Ligase Chain Reaction Amplification of Genomic DNA

Ligase Chain Reaction Mutation Detection

Utilizing Mutant-Specific
Oligonucleotide Primers

Wild-Type Sequence   Mutant Sequence

Annealing

Ligation

No DNA Products   DNA Product

LCR Detection of
Chlamydia trachomatis

- Cryptic plasmid target sequence (7–10 copies per organism)

- 48 bp target within the cryptic plasmid

- Unique DNA sequence (confers specificity)

- Highly conserved among all *C. trachomatis* serovars

Nucleic Acid Sequence Based
Amplification (NASBA)

- Reactions are isothermal (eliminating the need for a thermocycler).
- All enzymatic reactions take place concurrently (reducing the total time to completion of procedure).
- Provides exceptional sensitivity (10^9-fold amplification).
- Applications include detection of HIV and other viruses (hepatitis, HTLV, CMV).

*Available in kit form from
Organon Teknika (Durham, NC)*

NASBA
The Basic Procedure

- Hybridization of oligonucleotide-T7P primer to target sequence
- Reverse transcription with reverse transcriptase (generation of RNA:DNA hybrid)
- Digestion with RNase H

NASBA
The Basic Procedure *(cont.)*

- Hybridization with target-specific oligonucleotide primer (P2)
- Reverse transcription with reverse transcriptase (generation of double-stranded DNA)
- Generation of RNA transcript by T7 RNA polymerase

NASBA

NASBA Oligonucleotide Primer Design

T7 Promoter Gene-specific Sequence

5′ ■■■■■■■━━━━━━━━━━━▶ 3′

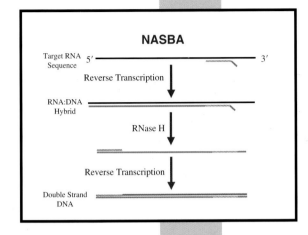

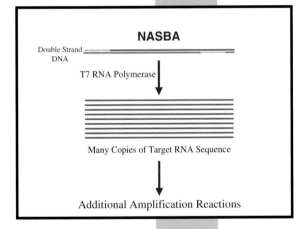

Transcription-Mediated Amplification (TMA)

- RNA transcription amplification system utilizes two enzymes (RT and RNA pol).
- Isothermal reaction, logarithmic amplification.
- RNA or DNA targets.
- Produces RNA amplicons.
- Hybridization protection assay (HPA) simultaneous detection.

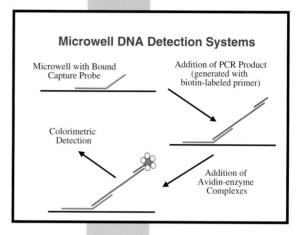

Microwell DNA Detection Systems

Microwell with Bound Capture Probe

Addition of PCR Product (generated with biotin-labeled primer)

Colorimetric Detection

Addition of Avidin-enzyme Complexes

Strand Displacement Amplification

Strand displacement amplification and homogeneous real-time detection are incorporated in a second-generation DNA probe system, BDProbeTecET.

Little MC, *et al.*
Clin Chem 1999;45:777–784

Strand Displacement Amplification
The BDProbeTecET System

This system is based on the simultaneous amplification of nucleic acids by SDA and real-time detection using fluorescence energy transfer. It is useful in infectious disease testing (*Chlamydia trachomatis* and *Neisseria gonorrhoeae*).

- **High throughput**
- **High sensitivity**

Strand Displacement Amplification
Instrumentation

The BDProbeTecET instrument is a fluorescent reader capable of maintaining constant temperature, monitoring real-time fluorescence, and reporting results through an algorithm.

Additional instruments include heating blocks for sample preparation and priming steps of the reaction.

Strand Displacement Amplification
Instrumentation

Priming microwell contains dried SDA primers, one dNTP, and fluorescent oligonucleotide probe.

Amplification microwell contains the remaining dried SDA reagents, including enzymes.

SDA Reaction Phases
• Target generation
• Exponential target amplification
• Detection

Strand Displacement Amplification
Target Generation

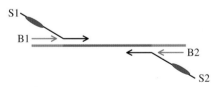

SDA Primers
B1, B2: Bumper primers
S1, S2: Single-stranded restriction enzyme site

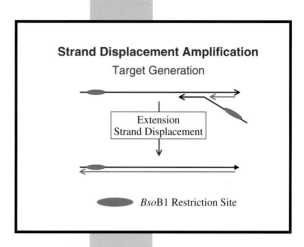

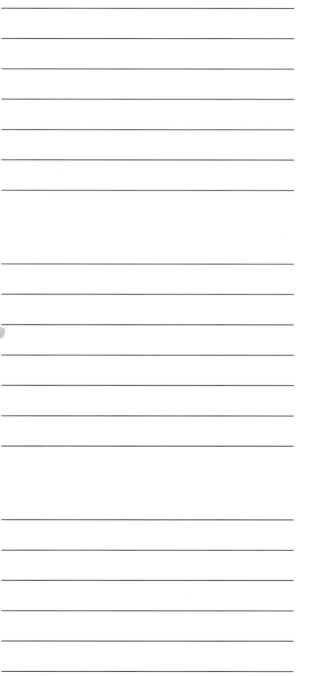

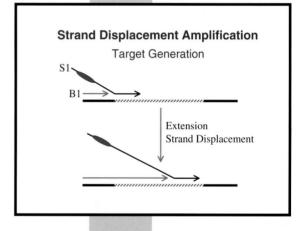

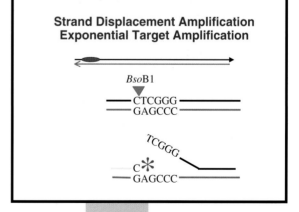

Strand Displacement Amplification
Exponential Target Amplification

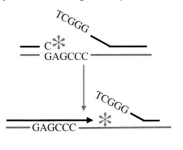

Strand Displacement Amplification

Mechanism of Fluorescence
Energy Transfer

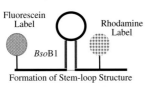

SDA Probe

Fluorescein
Label

Rhodamine
Label

*Bso*B1

Formation of Stem-loop Structure

Strand Displacement Amplification

Mechanism of Fluorescence
Energy Transfer

Fluorescein
Label

Rhodamine
Label

Dual-dye
Labeled
Hairpin Probe

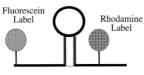

Cleaved Duplex
Yields
Fluorescent
Signal

*Bso*B1

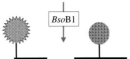

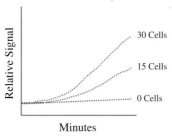

Strand Displacement Amplification

Detection of *Neisseria gonorrhoeae*

- 30 Cells
- 15 Cells
- 0 Cells

Relative Signal

Minutes

Branched DNA Detection

- Target nucleic acid sequences are not replicated through enzymatic amplification.

- Detection sensitivity is provided by amplification of the signal from the probe.

- Uses "capture probes," "bDNA probes" and "bDNA amplifier probes."

- Assay is based upon microtiter plate technology.

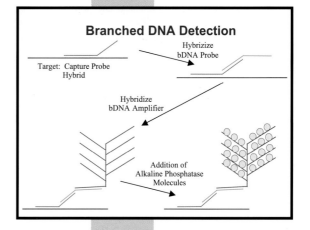

Branched DNA Detection

Target: Capture Probe Hybrid

Hybrizize bDNA Probe

Hybridize bDNA Amplifier

Addition of Alkaline Phosphatase Molecules

Blotting and Detection Techniques

Direct Detection

Scenario #1:
You know a patient has an infection with organism X. Several gene sequences are available for this specific organism.

How do you detect it?
(Note: known gene sequence)

PCR Amplification

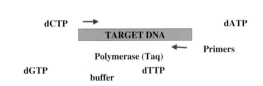

dCTP →   dATP
TARGET DNA
                                    ← Primers
Polymerase (Taq)
dGTP   dTTP
        buffer

Direct Detection

Controls

PCR amplification

↓

Gel electrophoresis   Gel type

↓

Gel stain

↓

Markers   **Fragment sizing**

Direct Detection

PCR amplification

↓

Dot/slot blot

↓

Probe hybridization 1. Isolation
2. Labeling

↓

Detection

Probe Isolation

- **Synthetic**

- **Cloning**

Probe Labeling

- End labeling

- Nick translation

- Random prime labeling

End Labeling

- Labeling of 3'-OH ends
- Terminal deoxynucleotidyl transferase
- Enzyme catalyzes formation of phosphodiester bond

LCx Semi-Automated Detection

MUP = 4-methylumbelliferyl phosphate

DNA Enzyme Immunoassay (DEIA)

Probe Coated Plate   Addition of Amplified PCR Product   Hybridization

Anti-ds DNA Antibody   Substrate

Direct Mutation Detection

Scenario #2:
You know a patient has genetic disease X. The gene for this disease has been identified and the mutation in this family has also been identified.

How do you detect it?
(Note: known gene sequence, known mutation)

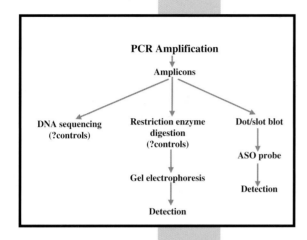

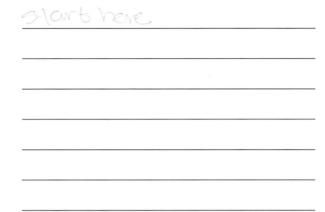

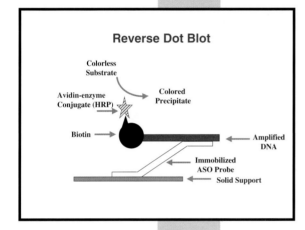

Screening Analysis

Scenario #3:
You know a patient has genetic disease X. The gene for this disease has been identified, but the mutation in this family has not been identified.

How do you detect it?
(Note: known gene sequence, unknown mutation)

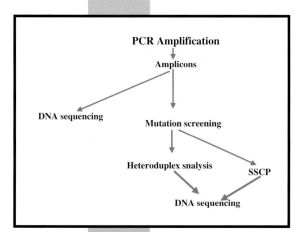

PCR Amplification

Amplicons

DNA sequencing

Mutation screening

Heteroduplex snalysis

SSCP

DNA sequencing

Heteroduplex Analysis (HA)

- Mutation screening method.
- PCR amplify region of interest.
- Mix normal and patient DNAs.
- Denature samples by heat.
- Slowly cool to room temperature.
- Add denaturing loading buffer.
- Electrophoresis on MDE gel matrix.
- HA fragments show retarded migration due to sequence differences.

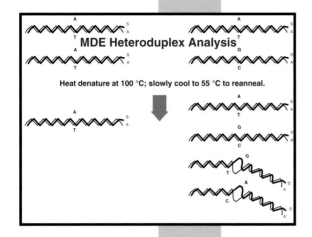

MDE Heteroduplex Analysis

Heat denature at 100 °C; slowly cool to 55 °C to reanneal.

Heteroduplex Analysis

Normal

Hetero-
duplex

Single-stranded Conformational Polymorphism (SSCP) Analysis

- Mutation screening technique.

- Short PCR products (<300 bp).

- Labeled amplicons for detection using small concentrations.

- Denature amplicons using heat.

137

_____

_____

_____

_____

_____

_____

_____

_____

_____

_____

_____

_____

_____

_____

_____

_____

_____

_____

_____

Single-stranded Conformational Polymorphism (SSCP) Analysis *(cont.)*

- Nondenaturing gel electrophoresis.

- Single-stranded DNA folds into three-dimensional shape.

- Different mobility due to different conformations.

Linkage Analysis

Scenario #4:
You know a patient has disease X.
The gene for this disease has not been identified and the mutations associated with disease have not been identified.

How do you detect it?
(Note: unknown gene sequence, unknown mutation)

Answer:
1. Linkage analysis
2. High throughput genomic screening

Microarray Analysis of Gene Expression

Three-color Comparative Analysis

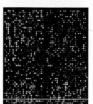

Microarrays Designs and Applications

cDNA Microarrays in Gene Expression Studies

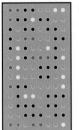

cDNA Microarrays
- cDNA clone inserts are printed onto glass slides at high density.
- As many as 25,000 cDNAs can be applied to a single glass slide.
- Enables large-scale, high-throughput analysis.
- Does not require knowledge of cDNA sequence.
- Thousands of known genes and ESTs are available.
- Requires special instrumentation for generation of microarrays and for analysis of results.

Complementary DNA Sequencing: Expressed Sequence Tags and the Human Genome Project

Adams MD, Kelley JM, Gocayne JD,
Dubnick M, Polymeropoulos MH,
Xiao H, Merril CR, Wu A,
McCombie WR, and Venter JC.
Science 1991;252:1651–1656.

Sample Preparation and Hybridization to cDNA Microarrays

Control Population   Treated Population

RNA Isolation

Fluorescent Tag   Reverse Transcription   Fluorescent Tag

DNA "Chip"   Mix and Apply to Array

Hybridize

Comparison of Gene Expression Patterns Between Normal Lung and Lung Carcinoma
for Identification of Genes Associated with Neoplastic Transformation

Normal   Tumor   Normal   Tumor

Patient 1   Patient 2

Comparison of Gene Expression Patterns Between Normal Tissue and Tumor Tissue
for Identification of Genes Associated with Neoplastic Transformation

Normal   Tumor

● Normal Expression Pattern
● Tumor Expression Pattern
○ Commonly Expressed Genes

Independent   Competitive
Hybridization   Hybridization

Comparison of Gene Expression Patterns Between Normal Tissue and Tumor Tissue
for Identification of Genes Associated with Neoplastic Transformation

● Normal Expression Pattern
● Tumor Expression Pattern
○ Commonly Expressed Genes

Housekeeping genes?

Tumor suppressor genes?
DNA repair genes?

Proto-oncogenes?
Tumor-associated antigens?

Comparison of Gene Expression Patterns
Between Primary and Secondary Tumors
for Identification of Genes Associated
with Tumor Metastasis

Primary   Metastatic
Tumor   Tumor

● Primary Tumor Expression Pattern
● Metastatic Tumor Expression Pattern
○ Commonly Expressed Genes

Independent   Comparative
Hybridization Analysis Hybridization

Comparison of Gene Expression Patterns
Between Primary and Secondary Tumors
for Identification of Genes Associated
with Tumor Metastasis

Genes associated with
neoplastic transformation?
Housekeeping genes?

Metastasis suppressor genes?
DNA repair genes?

Genes associated with
tumor metastasis?

● Primary Tumor Expression Pattern
● Metastatic Tumor Expression Pattern
○ Commonly Expressed Genes

Developments in
Gene Expression Profiling

- Quantitative monitoring of gene expression patterns with a complementary DNA microarray. Schena M, Shalon D, Davis RW, and Brown PO. Science 1995;270:467–470.

- Parallel human genome analysis: Microarray-based expression monitoring of 1000 genes. Schena M, Shalon D, Heller R, Chai A, Brown PO, and Davis RW. Proc Natl Acad Sci USA 1993:10614–10619.

- Use of a cDNA microarray to analyse gene expression patterns in human cancer. DeRisi J, Penland L, Brown PO, Bittner ML, Meltzer PS, Ray M, Chen Y, Su YA, and Trent JM. Nature Genetics 1996;14:457–460.

_____

_____

_____

_____

_____

_____

_____

_____

_____

_____

_____

_____

_____

_____

_____

_____

_____

_____

Microarrays Designs and Applications

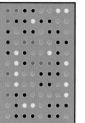

Microarray Probes
• cDNAs (from libraries or PCR products)
• Oligonucleotides
• Genomic DNA fragments

Applications
• Gene expression studies
• Oligo-mediated sequencing
• Genetic mapping studies
• Mutation analysis
• Polymorphism analysis

General Design of DNA Microarrays

Hybridization Standards

Gene Expression Controls
(Constitutive Genes)

Gene Probes of Interest

Development of a Toxicant Signature for a Known Agent or Agent Family
for Multiple Agents of
One Family Using an Index Cell Line

Agent A   Agent B   Agent C   Agent D

● Hybridization Standards
● Inconsistent Expression
○ Consensus Expression

Development of a Toxicant Signature
for a Known Agent or Agent Family
for a Single Agent Using Multiple Cell Lines

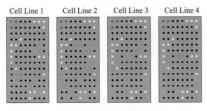

Cell Line 1   Cell Line 2   Cell Line 3   Cell Line 4

● Hybridization Standards
● Inconsistent Expression
○ Consensus Expression

Development of a Toxicant Signature
for a Known Agent or Agent Family

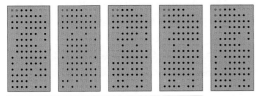

Raw Data   Consensus
Expression
Pattern

Development of a Toxicant Signature
for a Known Agent or Agent Family

Selection of Genes with Consistent Toxicant-
induced Expression Changes

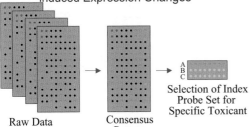

A
B
C
Raw Data   Consensus   Selection of Index
Pattern   Probe Set for
Specific Toxicant

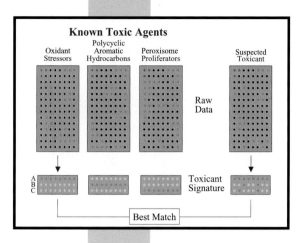

The tools provided to us by our understanding of molecular biology are what allow us to interrogate DNA/RNA for the purpose of identifying disease causing genetic alterations.

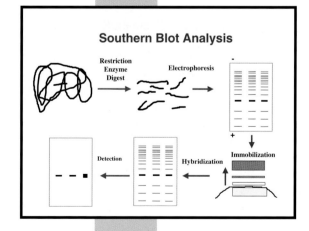

Southern Blot Transfer

- Vacuum or capillary action:
  - DNA is denatured *in situ* (in the gel).
  - DNA fragments transferred from gel to solid support.
- Large fragments transfer slower than small fragments.
- Gel treatment:
  - Depurinate with weak acid (reduces fragment size and increases transfer efficiency.
  - Denature with strong base, NaOH (hydrolyzes phosphodiester backbone at depurinated sites).

Southern Blot Transfer
(Pre-transfer Gel Photo)

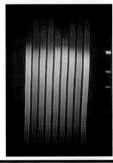

Southern Blot Transfer
(Post-transfer Gel Photo)

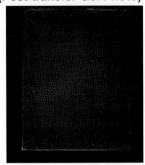

Southern Blot Transfer
(Post-transfer Membrane Photo)

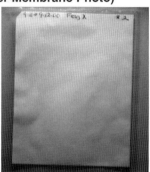

1. Bake or UV crosslink to fix DNA to membrane.

2. Prehybridization (blocking step to eliminate nonspecific probe hybridization).

3. Hybridization and detection.

Molecular Cloning

Genetic engineering includes techniques that allow for the construction of novel DNA molecules by joining DNA sequences from different sources.

Recombinant DNA
↓
Vector
↓
Clone

Characteristics of Cloning
Vectors

Vector	Insert size	Comments
Plasmid	<10 kb	Independent genetic unit from bacterial chromosome; consists of origin of replication, marker gene, promoter, polycloning site.
Bacteriophage	Approx. 25 kb	Selection based on size of insert and deletion of specific vector genes.
Cosmids	35–45 kb	Modified plasmids, packaged into bacteriophage.
Bacteriophage P1	Up to 100 kb	Capabilities between YACS and cosmids.
YACS	1–2 Mb	Yeast artificial chromosomes propagated as separate chromosomes in yeast; low efficiency and poor isolation.

Common Features of Cloning
Vectors

Multiple Cloning
Site   (HindIII PstI EcoRI SalI BamHI KpnI)
Polylinker

amp^r

ori

1. Replicator (ori)
2. Selectable marker
3. Cloning site

Cloning with a Plasmid Vector

Cloning Site

Plasmid

Restriction
Endonuclease
Treatment

Ligation of
Foreign DNA

Transformation
of Bacteria

Isolation of
Cloned DNA

Growth of
Bacteria

FRAX Syndrome Probe

- Probe name: StB12.3
- Locus: FRAXA
- Chromosomal location: Xq27.3
- Vector: pBluescript II
- Resistance: Ampicillin
- Vector size: 2.9 kb
- Insert size: 1.2 kb
- Excision enzyme: PstI

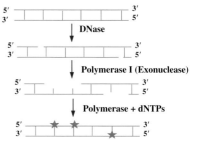

Nick Translation

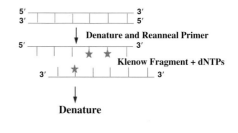

Random Prime Labeling

Prehybridization Blocking Reagents

- **Blocking DNA (minimizes probe binding to nonspecific sequences).**
  - Salmon sperm DNA
  - Herring DNA
  - Human Alu repeats
  - Human LINE-1
- **Blocking proteins (minimizes nonspecific binding of probe to membrane).**
  - Casein (milk protein)
  - Denhardt's solution (BSA, Ficoll)

DNA Hybridization

Hybridization is the formation of a duplex
between two complementary sequences.

1. Intra-molecular hybridization (ssLoop
    structures)

2. Inter-molecular hybridization

2/13/07

Stringency

Stringency includes the conditions of
hybridization that control the specificity of
binding between two single-strand portions
of nucleic acid (usually probe and
immobilized target sequence).

1. Increased temperature or decreased
    ionic strength (salt), increases
    stringency.
2. Only duplexes with near perfect
    sequence complimentarity can exist at
    high stringency.

Conditions for Hybrid Formation

- Temperature
- Salt concentration
- Concentration of nucleic acids
- Presence of denaturing agents (formamide)
- Presence of HMW polymers (dextran
  sulfate) increases [nucleic acids] by
  excluding volume.

_____

_____

_____

_____

_____

_____

_____

Stringent vs. Relaxed Hybridization		
	Temperature	**Salt**
Relaxed	lower	higher
Stringent	higher	lower

_____

_____

_____

_____

_____

_____

Detection Methods

Isotopic labels (^{3}H, ^{32}P, ^{35}S, ^{125}I)
1. Photographic exposure (X-ray film)
2. Quantification (scintillation counting, densitometry)

Non-isotopic labels (enzymes, lumiphores)
1. Enzymatic reactions (peroxidase, alkaline phosphatase)
2. Luminescence (Adamantyl Phosphate derivatives, "lumiphos")

_____

_____

_____

_____

_____

_____

Radioactive Labels

- ^{32}P: t1/2 = 14.3 days

- ^{33}P: t1/2 = 25.4 days

- ^{35}S: t1/2 = 87.4 days

- ^{3}H: t1/2 = 12.4 years

Southern Blot Analysis of Genomic DNA

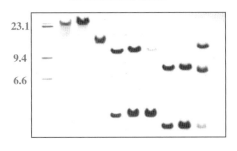

Factors Affecting the Hybridization Signal

- Amount of genomic DNA
- Proportion of the genome that is complementary to the probe
- Size of the probe (short probe = low signal)
- Labeling efficiency of the probe
- Amount of DNA transferred to membrane

Applications of Southern Blotting

- Deletions/insertions
- Point mutations/polymorphisms
- Structural rearrangements

---

4) transfer:

    a) capillary

    b) vacuum

    c) pressure

immobilize → block

5) hybridization

*detects mutation
* gives speci info about isolated product

Southern Blot Analysis of Insertion Sequences

5.5 kb

Probe

6.5 kb

Probe

Southern Blot Analysis of Insertion Sequences

1. Extract DNA
2. Digest with restriction enzyme
3. Gel electrophoresis
4. Transfer
5. Hybridization
6. Detection

7 kb
6 kb
5 kb
4 kb
3 kb
2 kb

Southern Blot Analysis of Polymorphisms (Linkage Analysis)

DNA

Probe

6 kb   4 kb

Invariant   Polymorphic Cut Site (1)   Invariant

0   (10 kb)

1   (6 kb)

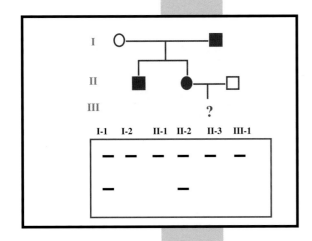

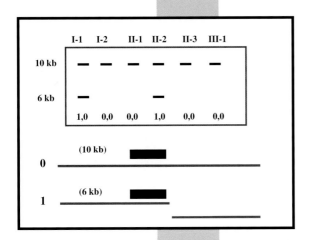

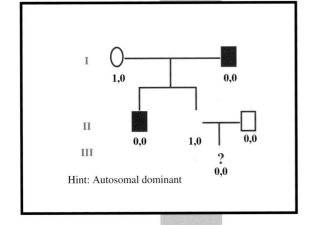

Hint: Autosomal dominant

Southern Blot Analysis of Point Mutations

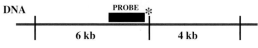

DNA

PROBE

6 kb   4 kb

If the mutation creates a restriction site, the probe will detect a 6-kb fragment in the mutant and a 10-kb normal fragment.

If the mutation destroys a restriction site, the probe will detect a 10-kb fragment in the mutant and a 6-kb normal fragment.

Detecting Large Structural Rearrangements

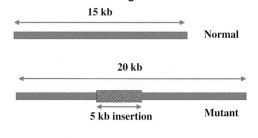

15 kb

Normal

20 kb

5 kb insertion   Mutant

Detecting Large Structural Rearrangements

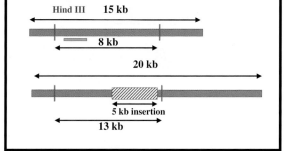

Hind III   15 kb

8 kb

20 kb

5 kb insertion

13 kb

154

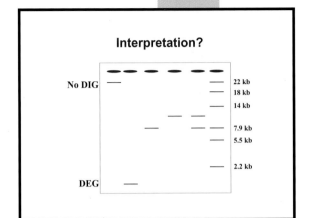

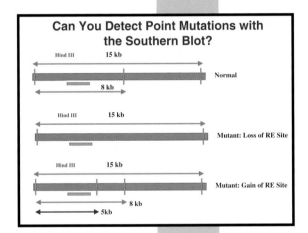

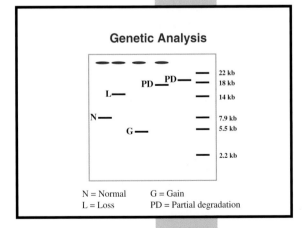

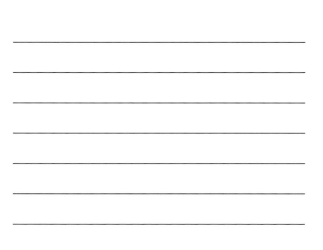

Sizing of Small Fragments Can Be Performed Using the PCR

150 bp — Normal
200 bp — Mutant
50 bp insertion
1. Single fragment
2. VNTR
3. STR

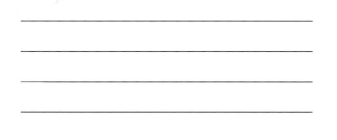

PCR Analysis of Small Insertions

150 bp — Normal
200 bp — Mutant
50 bp insertion

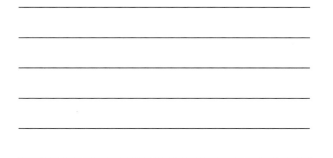

Can the PCR Be Used for Detection of Point Mutations?

Hind III 150 bp
80 bp
Hind III 150 bp — Amplimer / Amplicon
Hind III 150 bp
80 bp
50 bp

Gel Analysis

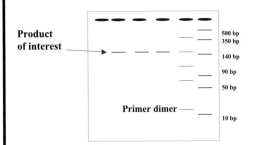

Product of interest →

	500 bp
	350 bp
	140 bp
	90 bp
	50 bp

Primer dimer —

10 bp

DNA Sequencing

While advances in molecular technologies continue to progress, DNA sequencing remains the "gold standard" for mutation detection.

What is DNA Sequencing?

DNA sequencing is the ability to determine nucleotide sequences of DNA molecules.

DNA Sequencing

- Gold standard for mutation detection
- Gold standard for histocompatibility typing
- Manual vs. automated methods
- Uses high-resolution denaturing polyacrylamide gels
- Resolution of large fragments of ssDNA that differ by a single base

Clinical Applications of DNA Sequencing

- Mutation detection
- Confirmation of mutation detection by other method
- Resistance testing
- HLA genotyping

DNA Sequencing Methods

- Technology
  - Chain termination
  - Cycle sequencing
- Chemistry
  - Maxam and Gilbert
  - Sanger
- Platform
  - Manual
  - Automated

Maxam and Gilbert DNA Sequencing

- Chemical cleavage of specific bases

- Piperidine cleavage of phosphate backbone

- Fragment size analysis by gel electrophoresis

- Not commonly used

Sanger (Dideoxy) DNA Sequencing

- Incorporation of 2′,3′-dideoxynucleotides by DNA polymerase

- Termination of elongation reaction

- Fragment size analysis (manual vs. automated)
  - Gel
  - Capillary

DNA Sequencing

Dideoxy (Sanger) Sequencing (ddNTP)

$^5CH_2OH$ O   OH
$_4$ C C_1
H   H
$_3$C C_2
H   H

2,3-dideoxyribose

3/20/07

3′ position
- missing an oxygen
- can't attach next nucleotide

deoxy (d)
dideoxy (dd)
nothing can be added to it
chain termination - sanger

159

random occurence

read sequence from bottom top
like a ladder.   bottom

start using a flurochrome to label
L7hit w/ light energy
becomes excited
& emits at a diff λ

can even label- A one color ⊕ new color
T diff. color C - new color

Dideoxy or Sanger DNA Sequencing

A	T	G	C
A	AT	ATTAG	ATTAGAC
ATTA	ATT	ATTAGACG	
ATTAGA	ATTAGACGT		

ATTAGACGT

ATTAGA
ATTA
A

A T G C

DNA Sequencing Detection Strategies

isotope / phosphor

- Labeled primer (starts rxn)
- Labeled dideoxynucleotide
  - Less background
  - No need for labeling multiple primers
- Fluorescent vs. radioactive

Clinical Scenario:
You know a patient has genetic disease X. The gene for this disease has been identified, but the mutation in this family has not been identified.

How do you detect it?
(Note: known gene sequence, unknown mutation)

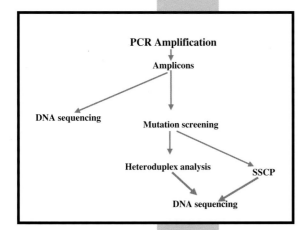

PCR Amplification

Amplicons

DNA sequencing   Mutation screening

Heteroduplex analysis   SSCP

DNA sequencing

Fluorescent *in situ* Hybridization (FISH)

- Probe (labeled DNA fragment)
- Metaphase chromosome spreads and interphase (nondividiing) cells
- Denature cellular DNA
- Hybridization
- Wash and detect

While classical cytogenetics requires actively dividing cells . . .

Cell culture
↓
Colchicine (disrupts mitotic spindle)
↓
Cells arrested in metaphase
↓
Cells lysed on slide
↓
Metaphase spread

... FISH offers the advantage
of being able to examine
nondividing cells.

Advantages of FISH

- FISH does not require mitotic cells (decreased TAT).

- Large number of cells may be scored.

- Dual color allows for simultaneous detection of multiple targets.

- FISH includes many sample types, including paraffin embedded tissues.

Importance of Being Able to Examine Different Cell Populations

- Some tissue types are difficult to grow in culture, thus low mitotic index.

- Some tissues are heterogeneous (contain more than one population of cells) that can grow at different rates.

FISH Probes

- Painting probes (cover all or part of a chromosome
  - Identification of marker chromosomes found in karyotyping
  - Confirmation of translocations

FISH Probes *(cont.)*

- Alpha satellite probes (identify centromeres)
  - Identification of marker chromosomes
  - Documentation of loss or gain of chromosomes (trisomies)

- Single copy probes (identify specific regions on a chromosome)
  - Used to determine presence or absence of a chromosome region

Single Copy Probes

- Used to count the number of copies of critical region of chromosome
- Probe cocktails = mixtures of >2 probes
  - One probe detects area of interest (single copy).
  - A second probe acts as internal control for chromosome number (alpha satellite).
- For translocations, two single copy probes used

FISH Detection

- Digoxigenin labeled probes
  - Antibody A (rhodamine or FITC labeled anti-digoxigenin)
  - Antibody B (anti-A)
  - Antibody C (rhodamine or FITC labeled anti-B)
- Fluorescein detection
  - Biotin-labeled probe
  - FITC-avidin or Texas red-avidin
  - Avidin/biotin antibody complex

Applications of FISH

Chromosome paints:
- Alpha-satellites
- Wolf-Hirschhorn syndrome
- Williams syndrome
- Prader-Willi syndrome
- Angelman syndrome
- DiGeorge syndrome/velo-cardio-facial syndrome
- Miller-Dieker syndrome
- Smith-Magenis syndrome

Applications of FISH *(cont.)*

Chromosome paints:
- Kallmann syndrome/steroid sulfatase deficiency
- Retinoblastoma
- Major ber/abi rearrangement t(9;22)
- Minor ber/abi rearrangement t(9;22)
- Translocation t(15;17) for acute promyelocytic
- Inversion (16) inv(p13q22) for acute myelomonocytic leukemia

SECTION

Molecular Diagnostic Testing

Goal

To introduce important concepts and considerations related to testing variables and quality assurance in molecular diagnostic testing, including pre-analytic and analytic variables, results reporting, and data interpretation.

Outline

- Quality assurance
- Pre-analytic variables
- Analytic variables
- Results reporting
- Interpretation of testing results
- Direct and indirect testing

Quality Assurance in Molecular Diagnostic Testing

A broad spectrum of plans, policies, and procedures provide a structure for the laboratory's effort to achieve quality goals (high quality analysis).

Quality control refers to those techniques that monitor performance parameters.

Testing Variables

Pre-analytical

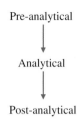

Analytical

Post-analytical

Molecular Diagnostic Testing
Pre-analytical Variables

- Test requests/ordering
- Patient identification
- Specimen acquisition, transport, and processing
- Preparation of work lists and logs
- Maintenance records

Molecular Diagnostic Testing
Analytical Variables

- Methodology
- Procedures
- Monitoring of laboratory equipment
- Monitoring of laboratory materials

_3/27/07_

start here

Molecular Diagnostic Testing

Post-analytical Variables

- Reporting results
- Interpreting results

**Pre-analytical Variables
In Molecular Diagnostic Testing**

Test Request/Ordering

Several variables related to test requests/ordering can significantly affect the quality of patient testing in the molecular diagnostics laboratory:
- Ordering an inappropriate test (desired test not performed)
- Illegible handwriting on an order (desired test not performed)
- Incorrect patient identification (testing performed on incorrect specimen)

**Pre-analytical Variables
in Molecular Diagnostic Testing**

Specimen Acquisition

Several variables related to patient specimen acquisition can significantly affect the quality of patient testing in the molecular diagnostics laboratory:
- Incorrect tube or container (testing performed on incorrect specimen)
- Incorrect patient identification (testing performed on incorrect specimen)

Pre-analytical Variables
in Molecular Diagnostic Testing

Specimen Acquisition *(cont.)*

Additional variables related to patient specimen
acquisition that can significantly affect the quality of
patient testing in the molecular diagnostics
laboratory:

- Inadequate specimen volume or size (desired
  testing cannot be performed due to lack of material)
- Invalid specimen (hemolyzed, heparin) (desired
  testing cannot be performed due to condition of specimen)
- Improper specimen transport (desired testing
  cannot be performed due to condition of specimen)

Analytical Variables in
Molecular Diagnostic Testing

- Quality of laboratory water supply
- Calibration of balances, glassware, and pipettes
- Temperature of baths, refrigerators, freezers,
  thermocyclers, and centrifuges
- Validation of methods
- Monitoring of technical competence
- Control materials
- Proficiency testing and accreditation

Possible Outcomes
of a Laboratory Test

- **True positive**: positive result for patients who
  have the disease
- **True negative**: negative result for patients who
  do not have the disease
- **False positive**: positive result for patients who
  do not have the disease
- **False negative**: negative result for patients
  who have the disease

169

_____

_____

_____

_____

_____

_____

_____

> **Molecular Diagnostic Testing**
> Considerations for Testing Validity
>
> _Sensitivity_ and _Specificity_
>
> - **Diagnostic/clinical**—based on outcome
> - **Analytic**—based on limit of detection and target specificity

_____

_____

_____

_____

_____

_____

_____

> **Molecular Diagnostic Testing**
> Considerations for Testing Validity
>
> **Diagnostic sensitivity**—the probability that a test for a specific disease will be positive
>
> $$\text{Sensitivity} = \frac{\text{True Positives}}{\text{True Positives} + \text{False Negatives}} \times 100$$

_____

_____

_____

_____

_____

_____

> **Molecular Diagnostic Testing**
> Considerations for Testing Validity
>
> **Diagnostic specificity**—when the probability that a test for a specific disease will be negative
>
> $$\text{Specificity} = \frac{\text{True Negatives}}{\text{True Negatives} + \text{False Positives}} \times 100$$

Pre-analytical Variables in Molecular Diagnostic Testing
Reporting and Interpreting Results

- Laboratory turnaround time
- Confidentiality
- Clinical correlation
- Client services/education

Molecular Diagnostic Testing
Direct and Indirect Testing Modalities

- Direct analysis—identification of specific genetic sequences or alterations/mutations (genotype) in nucleic acids isolated from a specimen corresponding to a particular disease/disorder (phenotype).

- Indirect analysis—does not identify the specific disease-causing mutation but determines whether the patient has inherited a marker located in proximity to the gene associated with a particular disorder (linkage analysis)

Molecular Diagnostic Testing
Direct Testing Modalities

- **Southern Blot**

- **PCR-based Methods**
  Allele-specific oligonucleotide hybridization
  Restriction enzyme digestion
  Sequencing of PCR product
  Electrophoretic methods

_____

_____

_____

_____

_____

_____

_____

_____

_____

_____

_____

_____

_____

_____

_____

_____

_____

_____

_____

_____

Molecular Diagnostic Testing
Considerations for Direct Testing

- Gene sequence must be known.

- You may or may *not* need to know the mutation spectrum within that sequence (depending on specific methodology employed).

Molecular Diagnostic Testing
Considerations for Direct Testing

If you know the gene sequence and the mutation . . .

Patient DNA sample

Southern blot   PCR

ASO blot   Restriction enzyme digest

Molecular Diagnostic Testing
Considerations for Direct Testing

If you know the gene sequence but *not* the mutation . . .

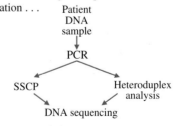

Patient DNA sample

PCR

SSCP   Heteroduplex analysis

DNA sequencing

Direct Analysis

Allele-specific Oligonucleotide Hybridization

Method employs normal-specific and mutant-specific
oligonucleotide probes in conjunction with high stringency
hybridization to identify allelic differences related to known
gene mutations.

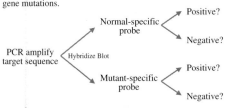

Direct Analysis

Allele-specific Oligonucleotide Hybridization

The most common mutation in Disease X, an autosomal
recessive disease, is located in exon 9 of the disease-
causing gene. This point mutation changes an A to G,
which results in an Asp to Ser substitution.

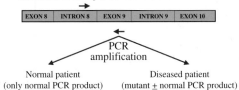

| EXON 8 | INTRON 8 | EXON 9 | INTRON 9 | EXON 10 |

PCR
amplification

Normal patient
(only normal PCR product)

Diseased patient
(mutant ± normal PCR product)

Direct Analysis

Allele-specific Oligonucleotide Hybridization

1 2 3 4 5 6

Normal Probe
Mutant Probe
ASO Blot

1 2 3 4 5 6

Normal Probe
Mutant Probe
ASO Results

Patients 1 and 4: No Mutation
Patients 2 and 5: Heterozygous Mutant
Patients 3 and 6: Homozygous Mutant

Indirect Testing Modalities

Southern Blot
- Restriction fragment length polymorphism analysis
- Linkage analysis

PCR-based Methods
- Microsatellite markers
- Linkage analysis

Considerations for Indirect Testing

Unknown gene sequence and/or mutation spectrum…

Patient DNA sample

Southern blot   PCR

Linkage analysis

Indirect Testing

Restriction Fragment Length Polymorphism Analysis

Method is based on Southern analysis of patient DNA that has been digested with restriction enzymes that reveal polymorphic variations in the genetic material. Segment-specific probes are employed to decorate the individual restriction fragments. Based on the pattern of restriction fragments, a patient allelotype is determined, which predicts disease probability.

Indirect Testing

Restriction Fragment Length Polymorphism Analysis

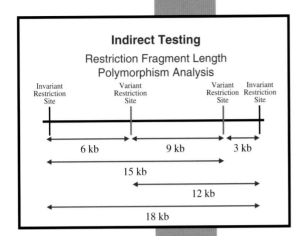

Indirect Testing

Restriction Fragment Length Polymorphism Analysis

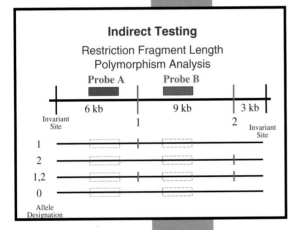

Indirect Testing

Restriction Fragment Length Polymorphism Analysis

Pedigree of two generations of individuals being tested.

I:1 — I:2

II:1   II:2   II:3   II:4

Indirect Testing

Restriction Fragment Length
Polymorphism Analysis

Southern Blot Results with Probe A

Family Member

I:1   II:1   II:2   II:3   II:4   I:2

Fragment Size (kb)

18
15
6

Indirect Testing

Restriction Fragment Length
Polymorphism Analysis

Southern Blot Results with Probe B

Family Member

I:1   II:1   II:2   II:3   II:4   I:2

Fragment Size (kb)

18
15
12
6

Indirect Testing

Restriction Fragment Length
Polymorphism Analysis

Family Member

I:1   II:1   II:2   II:3   II:4   I:2

Fragment Size (kb)

18
15
6

Probe A

Fragment Size (kb)

18
15
12
6

Probe B

0,2   0,1   0,2   2,1   2,2   1,2

Patient Allelotype

Indirect Testing

Restriction Fragment Length Polymorphism Analysis

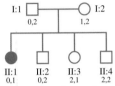

Disease X is an autosomal recessive disorder, where the gene responsible is proximal to one of the polymorphic restriction sites.

Indirect Testing

Restriction Fragment Length Polymorphism Analysis

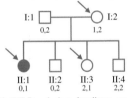

Based on this RFLP analysis and pedigree, we can conclude that the disease-causing gene is proximal to variant restriction site 1. Thus, patient II:3 may be at risk for the disease, and II:1 and II:3 will be disease gene carriers, like their parent I:2.

Molecular Genetics

4/3/07

Start here

Goal

To introduce essential concepts related to genetic diseases, including Bayes Theorem and the Hardy-Weinberg Law; to introduce common genetic disorders and provide examples of pedigree analysis of those disorders; and to discuss the role of molecular analysis of common genetic disorders

---

Outline

- Molecular genetic testing
- Principles of inheritance
- Types of genetic disorders
- Genetic risk calculation
- Hardy-Weinberg Law and Bayes Theorem
- Molecular analysis of common genetic disorders

Molecular Genetic Testing
Potential Benefits for the Patient

- Disease risk assessment
- Early detection of disease
- Disease classification/diagnosis
- Prognostication

Molecular Genetic Testing
Identification of Carriers of Disease Genes

- Early diagnosis of predisposition gene carriers
- Identify normal individuals to be excluded from frequent examination
- Identify unaffected gene carriers
- Prenatal screening

Molecular Genetic Testing
Implications of Predictive Testing

For the patient:
- Improved prognostication
- Determination of risks for other diseases

For the patient's family:
- Identifies other family members at risk for disease development

Molecular Genetic Testing
Predictive Testing

Advantages
Non-carriers
- Low risk
- Normal career
- Normal family planning

Carriers
- Increased medical surveillance
- Prenatal testing

_____

_____

_____

_____

_____

_____

Molecular Genetic Testing
Predictive Testing *(cont.)*

Disadvantages

Non-carriers
- Survivor guilt
- Testing error
- Have versus have not

Carriers
- Confusion
- Anxiety
- Depression
- Loss of job
- Loss of insurance

_____

_____

_____

_____

_____

_____

Principles of Inheritance

- From each chromosome pair, one chromosome is inherited from each parent (maternal and paternal chromosomes).
- Each individual has two copies of each chromosome, and therefore two copies of each gene.
- Meiosis reduces cells to only one copy of each chromosome.
- There is a 50/50 chance that each chromosome will be passed to the next generation.

_____

_____

_____

_____

_____

_____

Principles of Inheritance
Genetic Status

- Homozygous—identical alleles at a chromosomal locus
- Heterozygous—two different alleles at a chromosomal locus
- Compound heterozygote—two different alleles at two different chromosomal loci in the same gene
- Double heterozygote—two different alleles at two different chromosomal loci in different genes

---

Principles of Inheritance

Penetrance—proportion of individuals with a gene mutation who actually express the disease condition

Founder effect—high frequency of a gene mutation in a population founded by a small ancestral group when one of the founders was a carrier of the mutation

---

Principles of Inheritance
Mendel's Laws

- First Law: Units of inheritance (genes) are stably transmitted through generations.

- Second Law: Two members of a single gene pair (alleles) are never found in the same gamete.

- Third Law (independent assortment): Members of different gene pairs assort to the gametes independently of one another.

Types of Genetic Disorders

Single-gene disorders:
- Biochemical defects
- Metabolic disorders

Polygenic disorders:
- Congenital malformations
- Diabetes mellitus
- Cancer

Chromosomal disorders:
- Multiple birth defects

(handwritten notes) - no carriers

(handwritten) Affected - 50% chance given

Autosomal Dominant Disorders

- Dominant gene is located on an autosome.
- Affected individuals have an affected parent.
- Each child of an affected parent has a 50% risk of inheriting the abnormal allele.
- Unaffected individuals do not have affected children.
- Males and females are affected equally.
- Inheritance pattern is vertical.

Autosomal Dominant Disorders

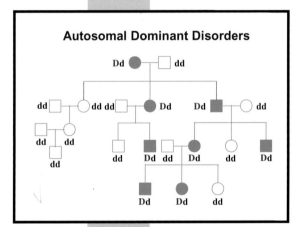

Autosomal Dominant Disorders

- Huntington's disease
- Neurofibromatosis types I and II
- Myotonic dystrophy
- Charcot-Marie tooth disease
- Familial hypercholesterolemia
- Marfan's syndrome
- Multiple endocrine neoplasia
- Retinitis pigmentosum
- Von Hippel-Lindau syndrome
- Adult polycystic kidney disease

Autosomal Recessive Disorders

- Recessive gene resides on an autosomal chromosome.
- Affect members of a family are usually siblings of the *proband.*
- Carrier parents have a 25% chance of having an affected child.
- Affected individuals may have unaffected parents (disease skips generations).
- Inheritance pattern is horizontal.

Autosomal Recessive Disorders

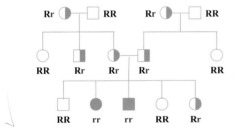

Autosomal Recessive Disorders

- Cystic fibrosis
- Tay-Sachs disease
- α1-Antitrypsin deficiency
- Gaucher's disease
- Sickle cell anemia
- Phenylketonuria

X-linked Recessive Disorders

- Affected individuals are primarily male.
- All female offspring of an affected male will be carriers of the disease gene (obligate carriers).
- Male offspring of affected men are always unaffected.
- Inheritance pattern is neither vertical nor horizontal.

X-linked Recessive Disorders

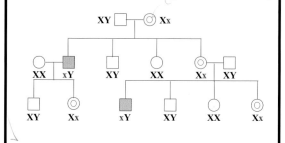

X-linked Dominant Disorders

- All female offspring of affected males will be affected.
- No male offspring of affected males will be affected.
- An affected female has a 50% chance of having an affected child.
- All affected individuals have an affected parent.

rare

X-linked Dominant Disorders

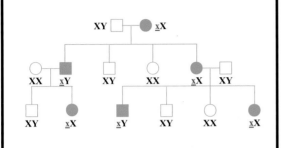

X-linked Dominant Disorders

- Hemophilia A
- Duchenne/Becker muscular dystrophy
- Fabry's disease
- Fragile X syndrome
- Spinobulbar muscular atrophy
- Lesch-Nyhan syndrome

Mitochondrial-associated Disorders

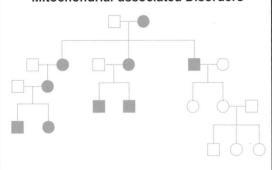

Mitochondrial-associated Disorders

- Leber's hereditary optic neuropathy
- Kearns-Sayre syndrome
- Mitochondrial encephalopathy, lactic acidosis, and stroke-like episodes (MELAS)
- Myoclonus epilepsy with ragged red fibers (MERRF)

Calculation of Genetic Risk
Rules of Probability

The probability (P) of two independent events (A and B) occurring at the same time is:

$$P(A \text{ and } B) = P(A) \times P(B).$$

The probability (P) of either of two independent events occurring is:

$$P(A \text{ or } B) = P(A) + P(B).$$

Calculation of Genetic Risk

- Two carrier parents of an autosomal recessive disease:

Rr × Rr

	R	r
R	RR	Rr
r	Rr	rr

1/4 (25%) = Normal
1/4 (25%) = Affected
1/2 (50%) = Carriers

Calculation of Genetic Risk

- One normal and one carrier parent of an autosomal recessive disorder:

  RR × Rr

	R	r
R	RR	Rr
R	RR	Rr

  1/2 (50%) = Normal
  0 = Affected
  1/2 (50%) = Carriers

Calculation of Genetic Risk

- Two carrier parents of an autosomal dominant disease:

  Dd × Dd

	D	d
D	DD	Dd
d	Dd	dd

  1/4 (25%) = Normal
  3/4 (75%) = Affected
  0 = Carriers

Calculation of Genetic Risk

- One affected parent and one carrier parent of an autosomal dominant disorder:

  Dd × dd

	d	d
D	Dd	Dd
d	dd	dd

  1/2 (50%) = Normal
  1/2 (50%) = Affected
  0 = Carriers

Non-Mendelian Inheritance Patterns

- **First**: Units of inheritance (genes) are stably transmitted through generations.
- **Second**: Two members of a single gene pair (alleles) are never found in the same gamete.
- **Third** (independent assortment): Members of different gene pairs assort to the gametes independently of one another.

- **First**: Some genes are unstable and can change from one generation to the next (premutation).
- **Second**: Two members of a single gene pair can be found in the same gamete (uniparental disomy).
- **Third**: Independent assortment is violated by genes closely linked on the same chromosome.

Non-Mendelian Inheritance

First: Some genes are unstable and can change from one generation to the next (premutation).

- Fragile X syndrome and other tri-nucleotide repeat disorders.

Non-Mendelian Inheritance

Second: Two members of a single gene pair can be found in the same gamete (uniparental disomy).
- **Imprinting**: differential expression of genetic material depending on whether it is maternal or paternal derived.
- **Angelman syndrome**: Deletion or mutation of maternal chromosome 15. Failure to express maternal 15.
- **Prader-Willi syndrome**: Deletion or mutation of paternal 15. Failure to express paternal 15.

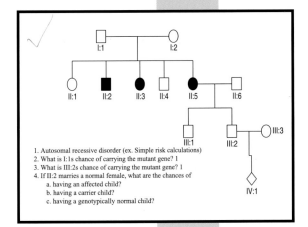

1. Autosomal recessive disorder (ex. Simple risk calculations)
2. What is I:1s chance of carrying the mutant gene? 1
3. What is III:2s chance of carrying the mutant gene? 1
4. If II:2 marries a normal female, what are the chances of
    a. having an affected child?
    b. having a carrier child?
    c. having a genotypically normal child?

Hardy-Weinberg Law

p =   frequency of normal allele

q =   frequency of disease allele

$p + q$ = 1 (assumes only two alleles)

p^2 = frequency of homozygous normal
       individuals

$2pq$ = frequency of heterozygotes

q^2 = frequency of homozygous mutants

$p^2 + 2pq + q^2 = 1$

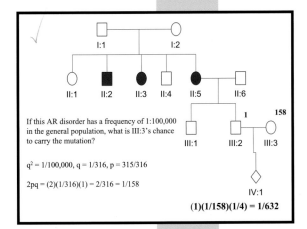

If this AR disorder has a frequency of 1:100,000 in the general population, what is III:3's chance to carry the mutation?

$q^2 = 1/100,000$, $q = 1/316$, $p = 315/316$

$2pq = (2)(1/316)(1) = 2/316 = 1/158$

$(1)(1/158)(1/4) = 1/632$

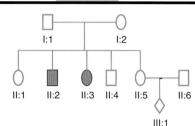

The general population incidence of this AR disease is 1:1600.
• What is II:5's chance to carry the mutant gene? 2/3

	R	r
R	RR	Rr
r	Rr	rr

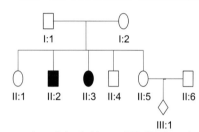

The general population incidence of this AR disease is 1L:600.
• What is II:6's chance to carry the mutant gene?

$q^2 = 1/1600$, $q = 1/40$, $p = 39/40$
$2pq = (2)(1/40)(39/40) = 39/800 = 1/20$

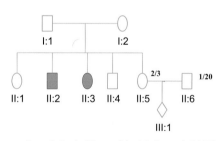

The general population incidence of the AR disease is 1:1600.
• What is III:1's chance to be affected with this disease?

(2/3)(1/20)(1/4) = 1/120

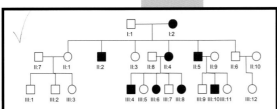

Autosomal Dominant
1. Affected offspring have affected parents.
2. Each child of an affected parent has a 50% chance of being affected.
3. Unaffected parents do not usually have affected offspring.
4. Males/females affected equally.
5. Vertical line.

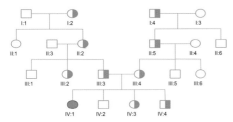

Autosomal Recessive
1. Carrier parents have a 25% chance of affected offspring.
2. Males/females affected equally.
3. Affected individual has unaffected parents.
4. Both parents affected, then ALL offspring affected.
5. Horizontal line.

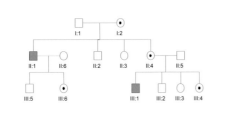

X-linked Recessive
1. Males affected most often.
2. Female offspring of affected males are obligate carriers.
3. Affected have unaffected parents.
4. Neither horizontal nor vertical line.

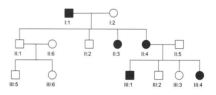

X-linked Dominant

1. All daughters but no sons of affected males are affected.
2. Affected female has a 50% chance for affected offspring.
3. Unaffected individuals have unaffected offspring.
4. Affected individuals have an affected parent.

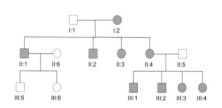

Mitochondrial Inheritance

1. Inherited only from the mother.
2. ALL offspring of an affected mother are affected.

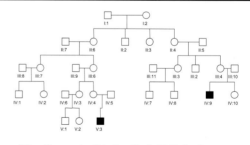

The disease in this family is X-linked

- Is it dominant or recessive?
- Who are the obligate carriers?
- Who are possible carriers?

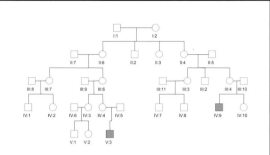

Only males are affected.
X-linked Recessive

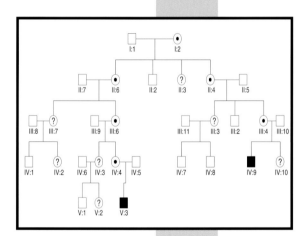

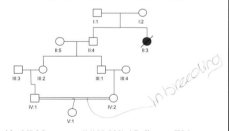

Individual II:3 has a rare (1/100,000) AR disease. IV:1
and IV:2 want to know the chance that their newborn
daughter (V:1) will be affected.

Hint: Because the disease is so rare, ignore the fact that
people marrying into the family might carry the gene.

_____

_____

_____

_____

_____

_____

_____

_____

_____

_____

_____

_____

_____

_____

_____

_____

_____

_____

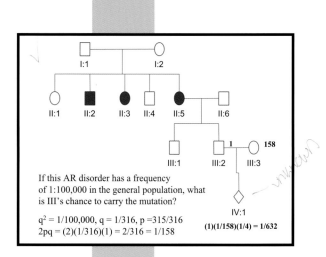

If this AR disorder has a frequency
of 1:100,000 in the general population, what
is III's chance to carry the mutation?

$q^2 = 1/100,000$, $q = 1/316$, $p = 315/316$
$2pq = (2)(1/316)(1) = 2/316 = 1/158$

$(1)(1/158)(1/4) = 1/632$

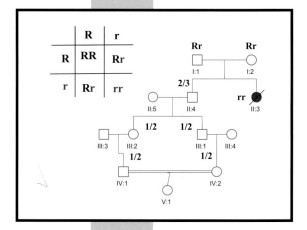

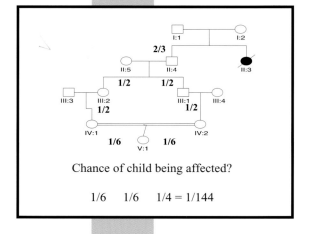

Chance of child being affected?

1/6   1/6   1/4 = 1/144

Bayes' Theorem

- Prior probability
- Conditional probability
- Joint probability
- Posterior probability

Bayes' Theorem

	Possibility I (carrier)	Possibility II (non-carrier)
Prior probability (Mendelian risk)	A	C = 1 – A
Conditional	B	D
Joint	A × B	C × D
Posterior	$\dfrac{A \times B}{(A \times B) + (C \times D)}$	$\dfrac{C \times D}{(C \times D) + (A \times B)}$

Bayes' Theorem

Conditional probability is the probability of observing a given condition. For example: Number of affected offspring, lab test results, etc.

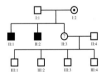

For an X-linked recessive disease, the daughter of a known carrier has a 50% chance of being a carrier. Is the chance lower for II:3 because she has 4 unaffected sons?

_____

_____

_____

_____

_____

_____

_____

Bayes' Theorem		
	Possibility I (carrier)	**Possibility II (non-carrier)**
Prior probability (Mendelian risk)	1/2	1/2
Conditional	$1/2 \times 1/2 \times 1/2 \times 1/2$ (assume person is carrier, this is the chance of having 4 normal sons)	1 (non-carriers will almost always have normal sons)
Joint	$1/2 \times 1/16 = 1/32$	1/2 or 16/32
Posterior	$(1/32)/(16/32) + (1/32) = 1/17$	

Thus, with 4 unaffected sons, chance is 1/17 not 1/2.

_____

_____

_____

_____

_____

_____

_____

Prevalence of Common Genetic Diseases

- Cystic fibrosis   1/2,000
- Tay-Sachs   1/4,500
- Sickle cell anemia   1/500
- AAT deficiency   1/3,000
- PKU   1/12,000
- Hemochromatosis   1/250

_____

_____

_____

_____

_____

_____

_____

_____

Sickle Cell Anemia
One Gene, One Mutation

- Sickle cell hemoglobin discovered in 1949.
- >400 human hemoglobin variants.
- Due to a single amino acid substitution in one of the globin chains.
- ↑ mortality/morbidity in Africa

Sickle Cell Anemia
Classification

- Sickle cell trait (AS): heterozygous

- Sickle cell disease (SS): homozygous

- Compound heterozygotes with Hb C and Hb D

Sickle Cell Anemia
Classification

- Sickle cell trait
  - Normal life expectancy
  - Hematuria
- Sickle cell anemia
  - Lifelong hemolytic anemia
  - Increased risk of infection
  - Variable course of illness

Sickle Cell Anemia
Molecular Pathology

- HbS differs from HbA by substitution of valine for glutamic acid at position 6 of the β-globin gene.

- Due to an A to T substitution.

- Intracellular fibers cause sickle cell deformity.

Sickle Cell Anemia

Normal (GLU)

CCT GGC GAG

Mutant (VAL)

CCT GGC GTG

How would you detect this mutation?

Sickle Cell Anemia

| Normal | CCT GGC GAG |
| Mutant | CCT GGC GTG |

M
N
RE
RE   RE

NM MM NN

N
M

Cystic Fibrosis

One Gene, Many Mutations

- Most common genetic disease in Caucasians
  - Autosomal recessive
  - 1 in 200 affected
  - 1 in 25 are carriers

Cystic Fibrosis
Clinical

- Clinically heterogeneous disease
  - Chronic obstructive lung disease
  - Colonization of airways by pathogenic organisms
  - Exocrine pancreatic insufficiency
  - Infertility
  - Increased concentrations of sweat electrolytes

Cystic Fibrosis
Molecular

- CFTR gene identified in 1989 (7q)
- 27 exons and spans 230 kb
- >700 mutations
- ΔF508 is most common mutation

Cystic Fibrosis
Phenotype and Genotype

Phenotype	Decreasing Severity of Disease			
Lung disease	Severe	Less severe	Mild	None
Sweat Cl-	Elevated	Elevated	Normal	Both
Pancreatic status	Insufficient	Sufficient	Sufficient	Sufficient
Vas deferens	Absent	Absent	Absent	Absent
CFTR mutations	Delta F508 G542X R553X	2789 + 5G > A R117H R334W	G551S R117H	F508C R117H

_____

_____

_____

_____

_____

_____

_____

Cystic Fibrosis

Molecular Diagnostics

How do you detect >700 mutations in a patient specimen?

1. Recommendations for a panel of 30–35 mutations (90%)
2. PCR/RFLP
3. Sequencing
4. Dot blot/reverse dot blot

_____

_____

_____

_____

_____

PCR-mediated Site-specific Mutagenesis (PSM)

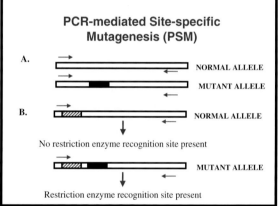

No restriction enzyme recognition site present

Restriction enzyme recognition site present

_____

_____

_____

_____

_____

_____

_____

PSM for Delta F508

Wild Type	Mutant
ATCATCTTTGGT	ATCATTGGT
ATGAT	ATGAT
ATGATCTTTGGT	ATGATTGGT
MboI	**No MboI**

Duchenne and Becker Muscular Dystrophy

- Most common form of inherited muscle wasting disorder
  - X-linked recessive
  - 1 in 3500 (DMD)
  - 1 in 30,000 (BMD)
- Slow debilitating disease
  - No therapy or cure
  - Onset of proximal weakness at 3 years old
  - Pseudohypertrophy of calf muscles
  - Progressive difficulty in walking

Duchenne and Becker Muscular Dystrophy

Molecular

- Dystrophin gene cloned in 1987
- 79 exons
- Spans 2.5 Mb
- Protein is missing in DMD
- Protein is truncated in BMD
- Major mutation is exon deletions

Duchenne and Becker Muscular Dystrophy

Molecular Diagnostics

- Deletion of multiple exons can be detected by:
  - Southern blotting
  - Multiplex PCR

_____

_____

_____

_____

_____

_____

_____

_____

_____

_____

_____

_____

_____

_____

_____

_____

_____

_____

_____

_____

Fragile X Syndrome

Phenotype

- Mental retardation
- Hyperactivity, autistic features
- Attention deficit disorder
- Speech impediments
- Long narrow face with prominent mandible
- Large ears
- Macroorchidism

Fragile X Syndrome

Genotype

- Expansion of trinucleotide repeat (CGG)

- Methylation of CpG islands

Fragile X Syndrome

Molecular Diagnostics

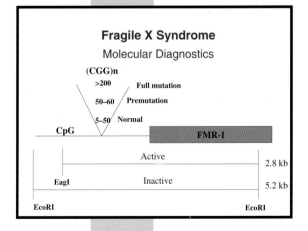

Fragile X Syndrome
Molecular Diagnostics

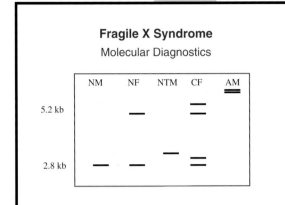

Fragile X Syndrome
Southern Blot Analysis

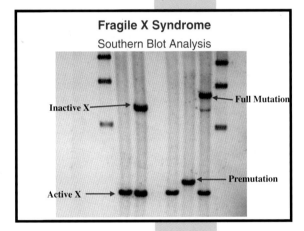

Fragile X Syndrome
Inheritance

- X-linked dominant with incomplete penetrance
  - 20% of mutant males are phenotypically normal
  - Daughters are asymptomatic with affected grandchildren
  - 30% of female carriers have some degree of MR

Fragile X Syndrome

Inheritance *(cont.)*

- Non-Mendelian inheritance
  - Lyonization
  - Anticipation ($\uparrow$severity, $\downarrow$age)

What about polygenic/multifactorial diseases that are quite common?

Hereditary Hemochromatosis

- Autosomal recessive iron overload syndrome
- Major defect: Excess gastrointestinal iron absorption
- Tissue iron accumulation causes dysfunction (liver, heart, pancreas, pituitary)
- Distinct from secondary iron overload or African overload

Hereditary Hemochromatosis
Clinical Symptoms

- Fatigue, 40%
- Liver Disease, 20%
- Arthritis, 20%
- Impotence, 40%
- Diabetes, 15%
- Pigmentation, 30%
- Cardiac Disease, 10%
- Asymptomatic, 30%

Hereditary Hemochromatosis
Diagnosis

- Clinical signs and symptoms are nonspecific
- Family history: HLA haplotype to affected relative
- Serum iron, TIBC, Ferritin
- Liver biopsy with determination of hepatic iron index
- **NEW**: Direct DNA detection of HFE C282Y mutation
- Quantitative phlebotomy
- Must exclude secondary iron overload

Hereditary Hemochromatosis
Lab Values

	HH	NORMAL
Serum iron (μg/dL)	180–400	60–180
TIBC (μg/dL)	250–400	200–300
Transferrin saturation (%)	>50	15–45
Ferritin (ng/mL)	300–10,000	20–200
Hepatic iron (μg/g)	5,000–30,000	300–2200
Hepatic iron index	>1.9	<1.0

_____

_____

_____

_____

_____

_____

_____

_____

_____

_____

_____

_____

_____

_____

_____

_____

_____

_____

_____

_____

Treatment of Hereditary Hemochromatosis
Phlebotomy

- Hereditary hemochromatosis is fatal if iron is not removed (cirrhosis, hepatoma, cardiac failure, arrhythmias, diabetes).

- Weekly venesections of 500–600 mL of blood for up to 3 years.

Treatment of Hereditary Hemochromatosis
Phlebotomy _(cont.)_

- One unit of blood removes 250 mg iron.

- Venesection every 3–4 months thereafter

- Iron chelators (Desferroxamine removes 10–20 mg/day.)

The HFE Gene

- Localized to HLA locus at 6p21.3

- C282Y (Cys→Tyr) mutation has high prevalence in hereditary hemochromatosis patients

- "G" to "A" transition

- Mutation creates an RsaI site

- Easily detected by PCR/RFLP assay

Clinical Utility of Hereditary Hemochromatosis DNA Test

- Confirm diagnosis of hereditary hemochromatosis.

- Replace liver biopsy as gold standard.

- Sensitivity = 80–90%.

- Specificity, 100%; dependent upon penetrance (number of individuals with mutation who will express the disease).

- H63D may also be associated with hereditary hemochromatosis.

Screening Hereditary Hemochromatosis

- Screen all adults with potential iron-related symptoms.

- Initial transferrin saturation test.

- DNA test to confirm and to replace serum ferritin or liver biopsy.

- IF DNA +, then follow annually with transferrin saturation and ferritin assay.

- Phlebotomy as therapy.

PCR-mediated RFLP Detection of HFE C282Y

| EXON 4 | Normal (C282) | Cys |
| EXON 4 | Mutant (282Y) | Tyr |

RsaI

C282   282Y   C282Y

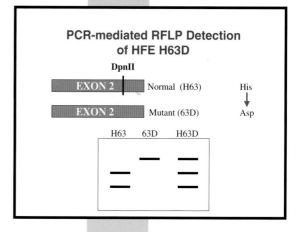

PCR-mediated RFLP Detection of HFE H63D

DpnII

EXON 2 | Normal (H63)   His

EXON 2 | Mutant (63D)   ↓
                        Asp

H63   63D   H63D

Hereditary Thrombophilia

- Pulmonary embolism results in 50–100,000 deaths annually in the United States.

- Hereditary deficiencies in proteins associated with coagulation predispose one to increased risk for thrombosis.

- Point mutation in the Factor V gene has been associated with increased risk of thromboembolism via APC resistance.

- APC resistance is most common cause of hereditary thrombophilia.

Risk Factors for Thrombophilia

- Circumstantial
  - Surgery
  - Trauma
  - Fractures
  - Complicated pregnancy
  - Oral contraceptives
  - Immobilization
- Genetic
  - Antithrombin III deficiency
  - Protein C deficiency
  - Protein S deficiency
  - Activated protein C resistance

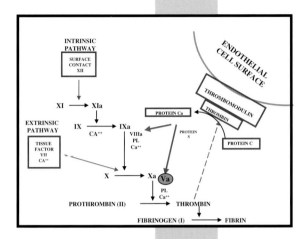

Activated Protein C Resistance

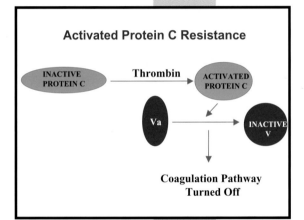

**Coagulation Pathway
Turned Off**

Activated Protein C Resistance

Normal Factor V
   . . . GAC AGG **CGA** GGA ATA . . .
              D   R   **R**   G   I

APC

Mutant Factor V
   . . . GAC AGG **CAA** GGA ATA . . .
              D   R   **Q**   G   I

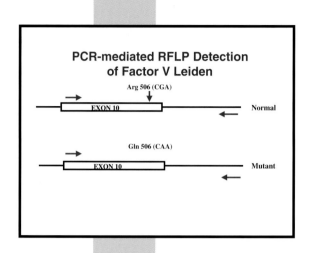

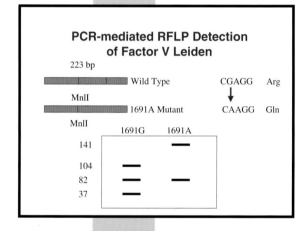

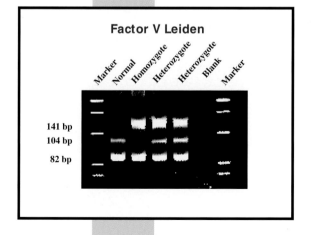

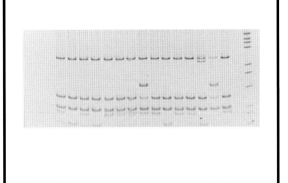

Genetic Alterations in Thrombophilia

| | PREVALENCE(%) | | | |
Defect	1st Event	Recurrent VTE	Normal	Risk
Antithrombin III deficiency	1	2–5	0.02–0.04	20–50
Protein C deficiency	2–5	5–10	0.2–0.5	7–10
Protein S deficiency	1–3	5–10	0.1–1	2
FV Leiden (APC resistance)	20	50	3–7	3–7 or 50–100
FII G20210A	3–8	15–20	1–3	2–5
MTHFR	10–20	10–30	5–15	2–3

SECTION 10

Molecular Oncology

_____

_____

_____

_____

_____

_____

_____

_____

_____

_____

_____

_____

_____

_____

_____

_____

_____

_____

Goal

To provide an overview of the cancer problem and to introduce essential concepts in cancer biology and multi-step carcinogenesis that impact on the identification of novel markers of human neoplastic disease and the development and application of useful molecular assays in the detection, diagnosis, and prognosis of human cancers.

Outline

- Cancer incidence and mortality
- Principles of multi-step carcinogenesis
- Oncogenes and tumor suppressor genes
- Mutational mechanisms
- Hereditary cancers
- Applied cancer molecular diagnostics
- Considerations for genetic testing

What Are Tumors?

Tumors are the result of a disease process in which a single cell proliferates abnormally, resulting in an accumulation of progeny cells.

The Genetic Basis of Human Cancer.
Vogelstein B and Kinzler KW (Editors).
McGraw-Hill, New York, 1998.

What Is Cancer?

Cancers are those tumors that have acquired the ability to invade the surrounding normal tissues.

The Genetic Basis of Human Cancer.
Vogelstein B and Kinzler KW (Editors).
McGraw-Hill, New York, 1998.

What Is Cancer? *(cont.)*

Cancer is a collection of diseases characterized by the uncontrolled growth and spread of abnormal cells.

Cancer Facts and Figures 1998.
American Cancer Society
www.cancer.org

Comparison of the Characteristics of Benign and Malignant Neoplasms

Benign	Malignant
Gross appearance	Gross appearance
• Smooth margins, encapsulated	• Rough margins, no capsule
• Center resilient, soft, viable	• Firm center, focal necrosis
Microscopic pattern	Microscopic pattern
• Resembles normal, well-differentiated compressed adjacent tissue	• Poorly differentiated
	• Invasive to adjacent tissues
• Intact basement membrane	• Disrupted basement membranes
• Cells and nuclei are normal size/shape	• Cells and nuclei are large/irregular

_____

_____

_____

_____

_____

_____

_____

_____

_____

_____

_____

_____

_____

_____

_____

_____

_____

_____

Comparison of the Characteristics of Benign and Malignant Neoplasms
(cont.)

Benign	Malignant
• Slow growth rate	• Rapid growth rate
• No metastatic disease	• Metastases are common
• Produces local effects	• Can cause local and/or distant pathophysio-logical effects

Cancer Is a Genetic Disease

• Cancer is a disease of genes or gene regulation that begins in a single cell and results in the loss of control of cell growth.

• Any cell type can become malignant.

• Carcinogenesis can result from acquired and/or inherited genetic abnormalities.

Cancer Represents a Group of Multifactorial/Polygenic Diseases

- • Environmental
  - – Chemical
  - – Radiation (UV)
- • Infectious
  - – Viruses (EBV, HPV)
- • Hereditary
  - – Germline genetic defects

Simple Questions About Cancer

- Does cancer represent a significant health problem for people?

- Who gets cancer?

- Are there any remarkable trends in cancer incidence or mortality?

Cancer Statistics

Publications

Hankey BF, Gloeckler-Ries LA, Miller BA, and Kosary CL. Overview. In: Cancer Statistics Review 1973–1989. NIH Publication No. 92-2789, I.1–17, 1992.

Landis SH, Murray T, Bolden S, and Wingo PA. Cancer statistics, 1999. Ca Cancer J Clin 1999;49:8–31.

Parkin DM, Pisani P, and Ferlay J. Global cancer statistics. Ca Cancer J Clin 1999;49:33–64.

Reis LAG, Kosary CL, Hankey BF, Miller BA, Clegg L, and Edwards BK (Editors). SEER Cancer Statistics Review, 1973–1996. Bethesda, MD: NCI, 1999.

Websites
http://www-seer.ims.nci.nih.gov
http:// www.cancer.org   http:// www-dep.iarc.fr

Estimated New Cancer Cases and Deaths

United States, 1999

Incidence, All Sites*
Total	1,221,800
Male	623,800 (51%)
Female	598,000 (49%)

Deaths, All Sites*
Total	563,100
Male	291,100 (52%)
Female	272,000 (48%)

*Except basal cell and squamous cell carcinoma of the skin

Cancer Facts and Figures—1999
American Cancer Society
www.cancer.org

The most common forms of cancer diagnosed are basal cell carcinoma and squamous cell carcinoma of the skin. Over 1 million cases of these skin cancers are diagnosed each year.

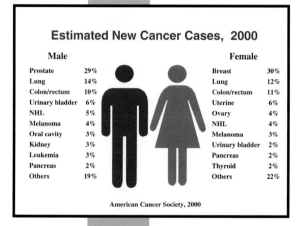

Estimated New Cancer Cases, 2000

Male		Female	
Prostate	29%	Breast	30%
Lung	14%	Lung	12%
Colon/rectum	10%	Colon/rectum	11%
Urinary bladder	6%	Uterine	6%
NHL	5%	Ovary	4%
Melanoma	4%	NHL	4%
Oral cavity	3%	Melanoma	3%
Kidney	3%	Urinary bladder	2%
Leukemia	3%	Pancreas	2%
Pancreas	2%	Thyroid	2%
Others	19%	Others	22%

American Cancer Society, 2000

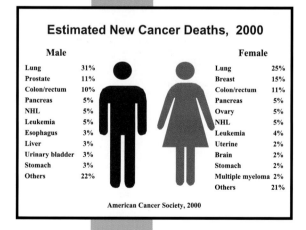

Estimated New Cancer Deaths, 2000

Male		Female	
Lung	31%	Lung	25%
Prostate	11%	Breast	15%
Colon/rectum	10%	Colon/rectum	11%
Pancreas	5%	Pancreas	5%
NHL	5%	Ovary	5%
Leukemia	5%	NHL	5%
Esophagus	3%	Leukemia	4%
Liver	3%	Uterine	2%
Urinary bladder	3%	Brain	2%
Stomach	3%	Stomach	2%
Others	22%	Multiple myeloma	2%
		Others	21%

American Cancer Society, 2000

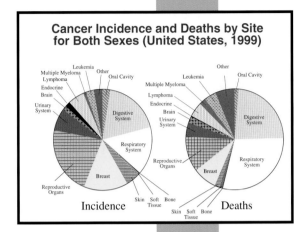

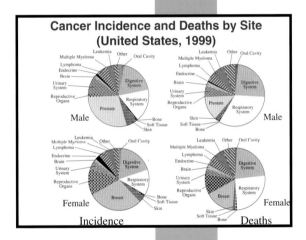

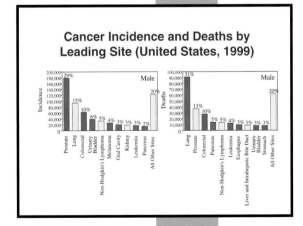

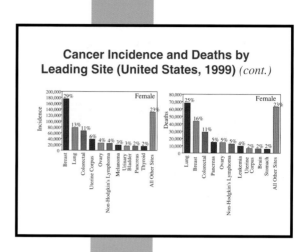

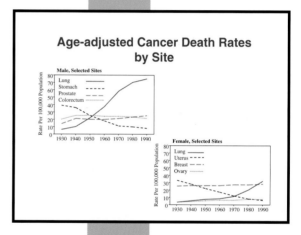

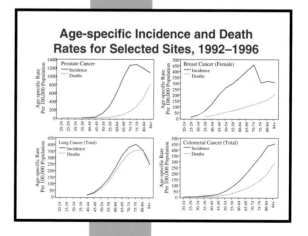

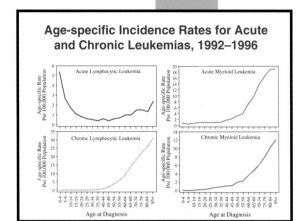

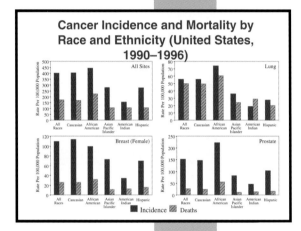

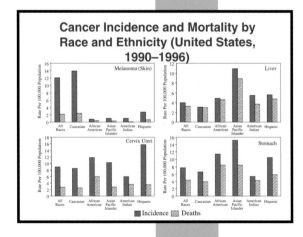

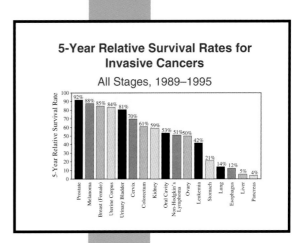

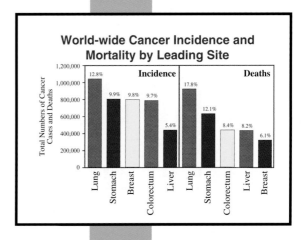

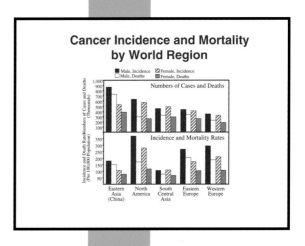

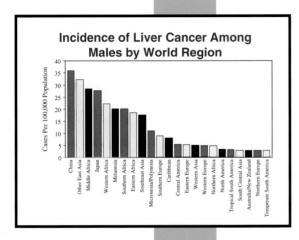

Incidence of Liver Cancer Among Males by World Region

Incidence of Prostate Cancer by World Region

Cancer Pathogenesis Involves Multiple Steps

Tumors are suggested to grow by a process of clonal expansion driven by mutation. The idea that carcinogenesis is a multi-step process is supported by morphologic observations of the transitions between premalignant (benign) cell growths and malignant tumors.

Foulds L. The natural history of cancer. J Chronic Disease 1958; 8:2–37.

Nowell P. The clonal evolution of tumor cell populations. Science 1976;194:23–38.

_____

_____

_____

_____

_____

_____

_____

_____

_____

_____

_____

_____

_____

_____

_____

_____

_____

_____

_____

_____

Cancer Pathogenesis Is a Multi-step Process

Normal epithelial cell $\xrightarrow{\text{Tumorigenesis}}$ $\xrightarrow{\text{Malignant transformation}}$ $\longrightarrow$ Carcinoma

Multi-step Cancer Induction with Chemicals Occurs in Definable Stages

Initiation $\longrightarrow$ Promotion $\longrightarrow$ Progression

---

Clonal Basis of Cancer Development

- Tumors arise from a single ancestral cell that has accumulated critical initiating mutations (genetic changes) and perhaps other epigenetic alterations.
- In some cases, these mutations (genetic changes) are present in all cells (genetic predisposition).
- Multiple mutations are needed for tumor formation.
- The number of mutations is independent of the tumor type.

Carcinogenesis Is a Multistage Process

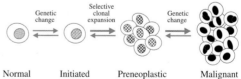

Harris CC. Chemical and physical carcinogenesis: Advances and perspectives for the 1990s. Cancer Res 1991;51:5023s–5044s.

Carcinogenesis Is a Multistage Process

Chemical
radiation
virus

Genetic
change

Selective
clonal
expansion

Genetic
change

Normal
Cell

Initiated
Cell

Preneoplastic
Lesion

Malignant
Tumor

Carcinogenesis Is a Multistage Process

Chemical   Endogenous
radiation   factors
virus

Genetic
change

Selective
clonal
expansion

Genetic
change

Normal
Cell

Initiated
Cell

Preneoplastic
Lesion

Malignant
Tumor

Carcinogenesis Is a Multistage Process

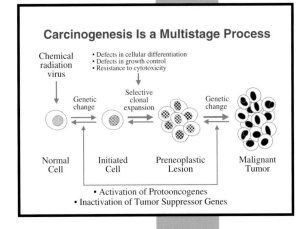

Chemical
radiation
virus

• Defects in cellular differentiation
• Defects in growth control
• Resistance to cytotoxicity

Genetic
change

Selective
clonal
expansion

Genetic
change

Normal
Cell

Initiated
Cell

Preneoplastic
Lesion

Malignant
Tumor

• Activation of Protooncogenes
• Inactivation of Tumor Suppressor Genes

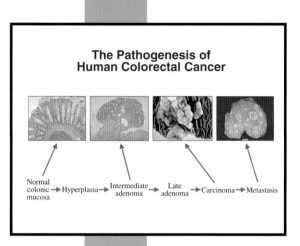

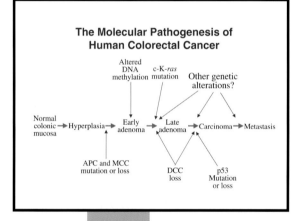

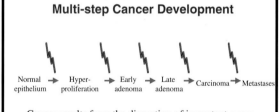

What Are Cancer Genes?

The classic definition includes cellular proto-oncogenes and tumor suppressor genes, as well as viral oncogenes.

The contemporary definition of cancer genes holds that cancer genes encode for positive mediators and negative mediators of neoplastic development.

Positive Mediators of Neoplastic Development

- Proto-oncogenes

- Growth factors and their receptors

- Metastasis promoting genes

- Cell cycle control genes

- Genes that promote cellular homeostasis

Negative Mediators of Neoplastic Development

- Tumor suppressor genes

- Metastasis suppressor genes

- Cell cycle control genes

- Genes that promote differentiation

- Genes that promote cellular homeostasis

Proto-oncogene and Tumor Suppressor Gene Products Regulate Cell Proliferation

Regulated by tumor suppressor genes   **Normal**

Proto-oncogene products → Cell growth and proliferation

Loss or mutation of tumor suppressor genes   **Cancer**

Oncogenes → Abnormal cell growth and proliferation → Neoplasia

---

The Cancer Gene Timeline

1911	Discovery of the Rous Sarcoma Virus
1970	RSV carries the *src* transforming gene
1979	Neoplastically transformed cells carry activated oncogenes
1982	Point mutations activate *ras* in bladder cancer
1983	Oncogenes cooperate to neoplastically transform cells
1986	*Rb* cloned, the first human tumor suppressor gene
1989	*p53* is a tumor suppressor gene
1993	HNPCC is related to defective DNA repair (mismatch repair)
1994	Breast cancer gene cloned
1995	*BRCA1, BRCA2*

Oncogenes

Oncogenes code for proteins that trigger cell division/cell cycle progression.

- Dominant acting/gain of function
- Qualitative change in oncoprotein expression

Growth factors (*sis*)
Growth factor receptors (*neu*)
Signal transducers (*ras, src, abl*)
Nuclear transcription factors (*myc*)

Functional Subcellular Localization of Proto-oncogene Products

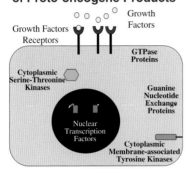

Growth Factors

Growth Factors Receptors

GTPase Proteins

Cytoplasmic Serine-Threonine Kinases

Guanine Nucleotide Exchange Proteins

Nuclear Transcription Factors

Cytoplasmic Membrane-associated Tyrosine Kinases

Genetic Mechanisms Resulting in Oncogenic Activation of Cellular Proto-oncogenes

- Point mutations
- Translocations
- Gene amplification

Ras Point Mutations

- Most common oncogene abnormality in human cancers
- *ras* genes code for membrane-associated proteins that trigger cell division
- Mutated ras proteins are stuck in the "ON" position

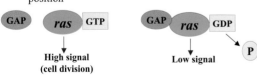

GAP *ras* GTP

High signal (cell division)

GAP *ras* GDP P

Low signal

_____

_____

_____

_____

_____

_____

_____

_____

_____

_____

_____

_____

_____

_____

_____

_____

_____

The c-*ras* Gene Family

- H-*ras*, N-*ras*, K-*ras*
- 21-kd proteins
- Active state contains bound GTP
- Inactive state (GDP)
- Hydrolysis of GTP to GDP is accelerated by GAP (GTPase-activating proteins)

Activation of the c-H-*ras* Proto-oncogene by Point Mutation

Normal c-H-*ras*

1	2	3	4	5	6	7	8	9	10	11	12	13		188	189
Met	Thr	Glu	Tyr	Lys	Leu	Val	Val	Val	Gly	Ala	Gly	Gly		Leu	Ser
ATG	ACG	GAA	TAT	AAG	CTG	GTG	GTG	GTG	GGC	GCC	GGC	GGT	...	CTC	TCC

↓

ATG	ACG	GAA	TAT	AAG	CTG	GTG	GTG	GTG	GGC	GCC	GTC	GGT	...	CTC	TCC
Met	Thr	Glu	Tyr	Lys	Leu	Val	Val	Val	Gly	Ala	Val	Gly		Leu	Ser

Mutant EJ-*ras*

Cellular Proto-oncogenes Activated by Gene Amplification

c-*myc*
- Leukemias, breast, stomach, lung, and colon carcinomas, neuroblastomas, and glioblastomas

c-K-*ras*
- Lung, ovarian, and bladder carcinomas

PRAD-1
- Breast and squamous cell carcinomas

mdm2
- Sarcomas

Cellular Proto-oncogenes Activated by Chromosomal Translocation Producing Aberrant Protein Expression

c-myc
- Burkitt's lymphoma and other B-cell lymphoma

PRAD-1
- Chronic B-cell leukemia

bcl2
- Follicular B-cell lymphoma

c-myc Translocation

- Proto-oncogene is removed from normal sequence-specific regulatory control mechanisms by chromosomal translocation

- Burkitt's lymphoma; t(8;14)

- c-*myc* (from chromosome 8) is translocated to IgH locus (on chromosome 14)

- IgH is a transcriptionally-active locus

- Translocation results in overexpression of c-*myc*

Proto-oncogene Activation by DNA Rearrangement

Promoter   1   2   3

Promoter X   1   2

Recombination

Promoter   1   2   3

Protein Overexpression

Chromosomal translocations may also
lead to the generation of fusion
transcripts that result in the synthesis of
a new chimeric protein
(such as bcr/abl or EWS/FLI1).

Proto-oncogene Activation by DNA Rearrangement

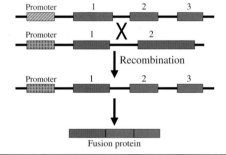

HER2/neu Gene Amplification

- Increase in gene copy number
- Intrachromosomal or extrachromosomal
- Results in increased gene expression
- Can predict prognosis or response to therapy
- Genomic versus proteomic detection may give different types of information
- Molecular analysis, cytogenetics, immunostain

Chromosomal Amplification

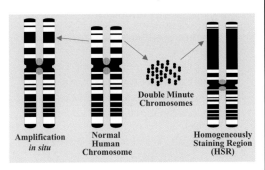

Amplification *in situ* — Normal Human Chromosome — Double Minute Chromosomes — Homogeneously Staining Region (HSR)

Tumor Suppressor Genes

Code for proteins that down-regulate cell division.

- Recessive acting/loss of function
- Expression inhibits cancer formation

Knudson's two-hit hypothesis of cancer development: Both alleles are inactivated by mutation or deletion.

Tumor Suppressor Genes or Their Protein Products Are Inactivated in Cancer

- One gene copy is mutated, while the other is lost (allelic deletion or loss of heterozygosity).
  - Most mutations are acquired (somatic).
  - Some are inherited (Knudson's hypothesis).
  - First hit (mutation) is inherited; second hit results from somatic mutation or loss (chromosomal deletion).
- Viral or cellular oncoproteins may also interfere with tumor suppressor protein function.

Tumor Suppressor Protein Functions

- Regulation of cell proliferation (cell cycle progression)
- Contact inhibition (cellular growth control)
- Signal transduction (cell membrane to nucleus)
- Gene expression (nuclear transcription factors)
- Cell cycle checkpoints ("guardians" of the genome)
- DNA repair ("caretakers" of the genome)

p53

- Located on human chromosome 17 at 17p13.3.

- Represents the most commonly mutated gene among all human cancers.

- Normal (wild-type) p53 protein localizes to the nucleus and has a short half-life.

p53 *(cont.)*

- Mutation results in abnormal accumulation of protein in the nucleus.

- After DNA damage, p53 functions to delay the G1/S cell cycle transition, enabling DNA repair.

- Wild-type p53 protein induces apoptosis.

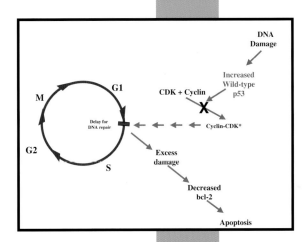

p53 Functions

- Induces the expression of proteins that stimulate DNA repair.

- Inhibits DNA replication.

- Induces apoptosis.

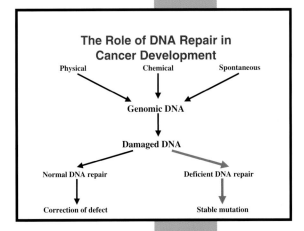

The Role of DNA Repair in Cancer Development

Damaging Insult

↓

Altered Oncogene or
Tumor Suppressor Gene

↓

Slow Repair or Early Replicating Gene

↓

Replication of Damaged DNA

↓

Transforming Mutation

Temporal Pattern of Gene Replication in Mammalian Cells

Telomeres

- Telomeres are repeated DNA sequences found at the end of linear chromosomes.

- In humans the telomere repeat sequence is (TTAGGG)n.

- At birth human telomeres are approximately 15,000 bp of (TTAGGG)n and this sequence shortens with each cell division by 25–200 bp.

- After approximately 100 cycles of reduction (shortening at each cell division), cells senesce (age) and can no longer divide.

Telomerase

- A ribonucleoprotein enzyme containing a complementary internal RNA component that is complimentary to the single-stranded overhang found at the chromosome telomere.

- Telomerase activity is found in germline tissues, stem-like cells, tumor cells, and other immortal cells.

- Telomerase activity protects and stabilizes (maintains) the integrity of chromosomal telomeres.

The Chromosome End (Telomere) Replication Problem

Telomerase and Cancer

Telomerase activity is expressed in many human tumors. Maintenance of telomere length inhibits cell senescence, resulting in cells with a distinct growth advantage and increased risk of acquiring new genetic alterations (chromosomal changes and/or nucleotide sequence alterations).

_____

_____

_____

_____

_____

_____

_____

_____

_____

_____

_____

_____

_____

_____

_____

_____

_____

_____

Molecular Diagnostics

The most significant challenge for molecular diagnostic laboratories is to establish clinically useful markers for multifactorial/ polygenic human diseases.

Guiding Principles for the Discovery of Novel Molecular Markers of Human Neoplastic Disease

Identification of novel molecular markers of human neoplastic disease will facilitate the development of useful molecular assays for detection, diagnosis, and prediction of patient outcome.

Molecular Diagnostics: Clinical Oncology

- Diagnostic

- Prognostic

- Predisposition

Molecular Diagnosis of Cancer
Effect on Patient Outcome

- Effective cancer treatment requires early detection of clinical tumors and/or effective monitoring of patients at high-risk for cancer development.
- Patients who present with clinically advanced disease demonstrate significantly poorer response to therapy and overall survival.
- Molecular diagnostics can positively impact on cancer detection, diagnosis, prediction of outcome, and risk assessment.

Early Detection and Patient Outcome

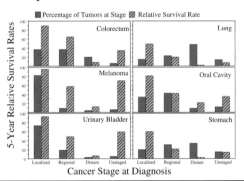

Early Detection and Patient Outcome

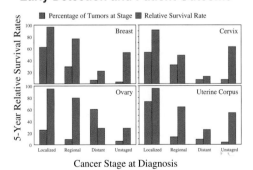

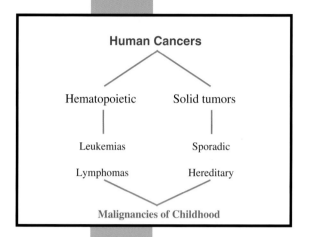

Human Cancers

Hematopoietic   Solid tumors

Leukemias   Sporadic

Lymphomas   Hereditary

Malignancies of Childhood

Cancer Predisposition

- Families displaying a high incidence for a particular type of cancer (such as Wilms' tumor).

- Families displaying a high incidence of several types of cancer or specific groups of cancers (such as those associated with Li-Fraumeni syndrome).

Cancer Predisposition *(cont.)*

- Families with a specific DNA repair deficiency who demonstrate a high incidence for a specific subset of cancers (such as those cancers associated with xeroderma pigmentosum).

- Family history is important for all cancers, including common types of cancer.

Characteristics Associated with Hereditary Cancer

- Multiple affected relatives

- Early age of cancer onset (clinical disease)

- Bilaterally affected organs (such as in breast cancer)

Characteristics Associated with Hereditary Cancer *(cont.)*

- Multiple primary cancers in the same individual

- Autosomal dominant pattern of inheritance

- Known associated cancers occurring in the same family (such as breast and ovarian cancers)

Cloned Cancer Susceptibility Genes and Their Corresponding Hereditary Cancers

Year	Gene	Location	Cancer
1986	RB1	13q14	Hereditary RB
1990	WT1	11p13	H. Wilms' tumor
1990	TP53	17p13	Li-Fraumeni syndrome
1990	NF1	17q11	Neurofibromatosis 1
1991	APC	5q21	Familial adenomatous polyposis
1993	NF2	22q12	NF2, Acoustic neuroma
1993	VHL	3p25	Von Hippel-Lindau, renal
1993	RET	10q11	MEN2, thyroid, adrenal
1993	TSC2	16p13	Tuberous sclerosis 2, renal
1993	MSH2	2p16	HNPCC
1994	MLH1	3p21	HNPCC
1994	PMS1	2q32	HNPCC
1994	PMS2	7p22	HNPCC
1994	CDKN2	9p21	H. Melanoma
1994	BRCA1	17q21	H. Breast Cancer
1995	BRCA2	13q12-13	H. Breast Cancer
1995	EXT1	8q24.1	Langer-Giedion, chondrosarcoma
1996	CDK4	12q13	H. Melanoma
1996	PTC	9q22.3	Gorlin syndrome, basal cell carcinoma

Li-Fraumeni Syndrome

- Familial cancer syndrome with underlying genetic susceptibility
- High incidence of childhood and adult tumors
  - Breast carcinoma
  - Soft tissue sarcomas
  - Brain tumors
  - Osteosarcomas
  - Leukemia
- Associated with germline mutations of the *p53* tumor suppressor gene

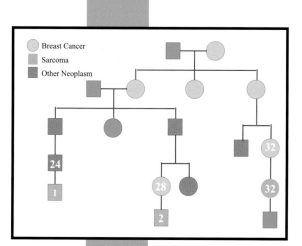

Breast Cancer
Sarcoma
Other Neoplasm

Retinoblastoma

- Intra-ocular tumor of childhood.

- Occurs in 1 of every 20,000 live births.

- Both hereditary and nonhereditary forms have been described.

Retinoblastoma *(cont.)*

- Inactivation of the *Rb1* tumor suppressor gene at both alleles is required for development of the tumor.

- 40% of retinoblastomas are hereditary, containing germline mutations in the *Rb1* gene that are transmitted as an autosomal dominant trait.

Hereditary Retinoblastoma

- Child is born with a germline mutation in the *Rb1* gene, resulting from an affected parent, a carrier parent, or a *de novo* mutational event.

- Tumor development follows the subsequent acquisition of a somatic mutation affecting the remaining normal *Rb1* allele.

Hereditary Retinoblastoma *(cont.)*

- Hereditary retinoblastoma is the prototype inherited cancer, the analysis of which led to the development of Knudson's two-hit hypothesis.

- Because of the significant risk to children, determination of whether retinoblastoma is hereditary (45%) or nonhereditary (0%) is critical.

The Two-Hit Hypothesis for Development of Retinoblastoma

- A. G. Knudson examined the frequency and age of development of inherited versus sporadic forms of retinoblastoma and proposed that the development of this tumor required at least two mutational events.

- The two-mutation model accounts for the dominant inheritance of a susceptibility to retinoblastoma. However, it was recognized that the susceptibility gene did not function as a single dominant determinant of neoplastic transformation at the cellular level.

Knudson Jr AG. Mutation and cancer: Statistical study of retinoblastoma. Proc Natl Acad Sci USA 1971;68:820–823.

Rb1 Gene Mutations

- The Rb1 gene is approximately 200 kb in size and contains 27 exons
- Frameshift mutations (most frequent)
  - Resulting from small deletions
  - Resulting form 1–2 bp insertions
- Nonsense mutations
- Missense mutations
- Splice-site mutations (least frequent)
- The majority of tumors arise from *de novo* (new) mutations.

Hereditary Retinoblastoma

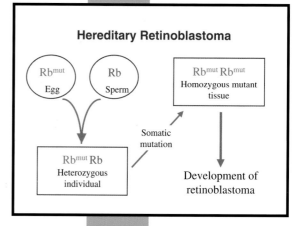

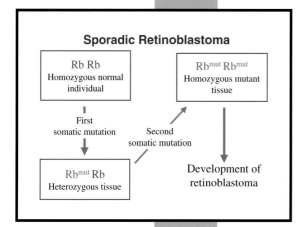

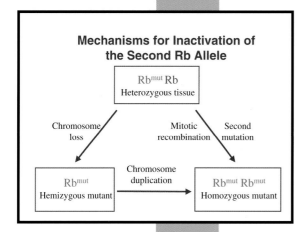

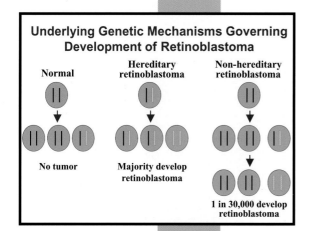

_____

_____

_____

_____

_____

_____

_____

Familial Colon Cancer Syndromes

- Familial adenomatous polyposis
  - Inherited loss or mutation of *APC* gene
  - 1% of all colon cancers
  - 100s–1000s of colonic polyps
  - Poor prognosis
  - 60% have *p53* mutations

_____

_____

_____

_____

_____

_____

_____

Familial Colon Cancer Syndromes
(cont.)

- Hereditary non-polyposis colon cancer (HNPCC)
  - Mutated mismatch repair gene
  - 3–6% of all colon cancers
  - Good prognosis
  - 25% have *p53* mutations

_____

_____

_____

_____

_____

_____

Familial Adenomatous Polyposis Coli (FAP)

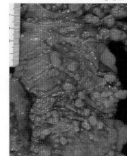

- Autosomal dominant
- APC gene (5q21) mutations
- Molecular diagnosis employs the *in vitro* protein truncation test (PTT)

Hereditary Non-polyposis Colorectal Cancer (HNPCC)

- Also known as Lynch syndrome

- Early onset colorectal cancer associated with cancer of the ovary, endometrium, stomach, small bowel, ureter, or renal pelvis

- Frequently involves germline mutations in one (or more) of several mismatch repair genes

- Accounts for 5% of all colon cancer

DNA Mismatch Repair Genes

Gene	Chromosomal location	Contribution to HNPCC
hMSH2	2p21-22	31%
hMLH1	3p21	33%
hPMS1	2q31-33	2%
hPMS2	7p22	4%

Amsterdam Criteria for Diagnosis of HNPCC

- At least three family members with colorectal cancer, two of whom are first-degree relatives

- At least two generations represented in cancer pedigree

- At least one individual younger than 50 years at diagnosis of cancer

Provisional Recommendations for Carriers of Mutations Associated with Development of HNPCC

- Risk of development of colorectal cancer is 68–75% by age 65

- Average age at diagnosis is 45 years

- Surveillance: Colonoscopy, every 1–3 years beginning at age 20–25 years

Provisional Recommendations for Carriers of Mutations Associated with Development of HNPCC *(cont.)*

- Surveillance: Annual screening for endometrial cancer beginning at age 25–35 years (transvaginal ultrasound, endometrial aspirate)

- Prophylactic colectomy in carriers of mutations with colon cancers or adenomas

Hereditary Breast Cancer

- 1 in 9 women in the United States will develop breast cancer, most occurring by age 70.
- 185,000 new cases per year in the United States and 43,000 deaths
- Approximately 5–10% are inherited or familial
- *BRCA1* cloned 1994
- *BRCA2* identified in 1995
- Inheritance of a BRCA gene mutation increases lifetime risk of developing breast cancer to approximately 85%.

Breast Cancer Risk Factors

- Age
- Family history of breast or ovarian cancer
- Early menarche, late menopause
- Smoking
- High fat diet

Detection of Breast Cancer

- Physical exam (self-exam)
- Mammography (tumors or calcified areas associated with a preneoplastic condition)
- Diagnosis is microscopic
- Most common forms of breast cancer are ductal and lobular
- Metastasizes to lymph nodes, lung, bone, brain

Treatment of Breast Cancer

- Surgical
  - Lumpectomy
  - Modified radical mastectomy
- Radiation therapy for local disease
- Chemotherapy for metastatic disease
  - Cytotoxic agents
  - Anti-estrogen therapy (Tamoxifen)

_____

_____

_____

_____

_____

_____

_____

Staging of Breast Cancer

- Stage I: <2 cm, no lymph node involvement

- Stage II: >2 cm but <5 cm or spread to lymph nodes

- Stage III: >5 cm

- Stage IV (inoperable): distant metastases (lung, bone, brain)

_____

_____

_____

_____

_____

_____

Women with Breast Cancer

- Early treatment of localized disease is best hope of cure.

  - Survival for stage I is 85% at 5 years, 65–75% at 10 years

- 2/3 demonstrate local tumor spread to proximal lymph nodes at the time of diagnosis.

_____

_____

_____

_____

_____

_____

Breast Cancer Susceptibility Genes
BRCA1

- Localized to chromosome arm 17q.

- Mutated in 45% of hereditary breast cancers and 90% of patients with breast/ovarian cancer.

- 120 different mutations have been identified.

Breast Cancer Susceptibility Genes
BRCA1 *(cont.)*

- Features of the *BRCA1* gene include 23 exons, and a large exon 11 (100 kb) that contains 60% of the coding sequence.

- Several families have been identified that contain individuals affected by breast cancer but lacking gene mutation, and others have been identified containing individuals with a mutated gene but no breast cancer.

Breast Cancer Susceptibility Genes
BRCA2

- Localized to chromosome arm 13q.

- Accounts for approximately 40–45% of early onset hereditary breast cancer.

- Mutation does not contribute significantly to risk for development of ovarian cancer.

- The *BRCA2* gene is 70 kb in size, containing 27 exons.

Prevalence of *BRCA* Gene Mutations in the Ashkenazi Jewish Community

BRCA1		*BRCA2*	
185delAG	1%	6174 delT	1.5%
5382insC	0.1%		
1294del40	0.02		
R1443X	0.01		
E1250X	<0.005		

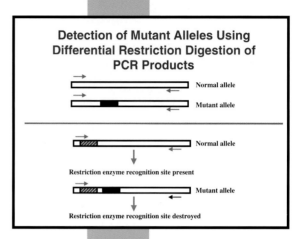

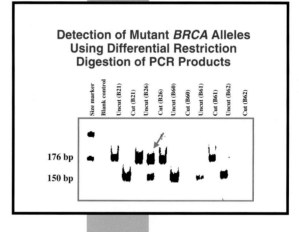

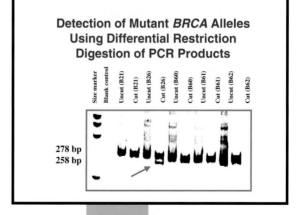

Chromosomal Translocation in Ewing's Tumor

- Small round cell tumor of childhood
  - Ewing's sarcoma (common bone tumor)
  - Peripheral primitive neuroectodermal tumor (pPNET)
  - Neuroblastoma
  - Rhabdomyosarcoma

Chromosomal Translocation in Ewing's Tumor *(cont.)*

- Microscopic classification of these tumors is difficult because the different forms share a similar histologic appearance.

- Tumor cells are uniformly bland, undifferentiated with low mitotic index despite rapid growth.

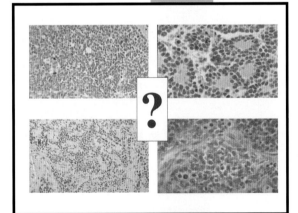

_____

_____

_____

_____

_____

_____

_____

Ewing's Tumors

- t(11;22)(q24;q12) occurs in 83% of cases.

- Translocation involves the *EWS* gene on chromosome 22 and the *FLI-1* transcription factor gene on chromosome 11.

- Translocation results in the c-terminal *FLI-1* coming under the control of the *EWS* gene promoter.

- Effective treatment and appropriate therapeutic approaches are based upon specific tumor type.

_____

_____

_____

_____

_____

_____

_____

_____

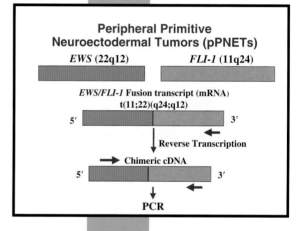

Peripheral Primitive Neuroectodermal Tumors (pPNETs)

_____

_____

_____

_____

_____

_____

_____

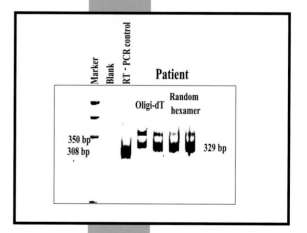

Translocations Diagnostic for Soft Tissue and Bone Tumors

Osteosarcomas	None
Extraskeletal myxoid chondrosarcoma	t(9;22)(q22;q11-12)
Tumors of connective tissue	
(fibrosarcoma, MFH, DFP)	None
Muscle tissue tumors	
Alveolar rhabdomyosarcoma	t(2;13)(q35;q14)
t(1;13)(p36;q12)	
t(2;11)	
Lipogenic tumors	
Myxoid and round cell liposarcoma	t(12;16)(q13;p11)
Ewing sarcoma and PNET	t(11;22)(q24;q12)
Desmoplastic small round cell	t(11;22)(p13;q12)
Clear cell sarcoma	t(12;22)(q13;q12-13)
Synovial sarcoma	t(X;18)(p11.2;q11.2)

t(X;18); SYT-SSX1 and SYT-SSX2

- **90% of synovial sarcomas**
- **SYT gene on chromosome 18**
- **SSX1 and SSX2 genes on X**
- **Can differentiate between spindle cell tumors**
- **Monophasic, SSX2**
- **Biphasic, SSX1**

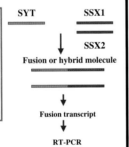

SYT   SSX1
       SSX2

Fusion or hybrid molecule

Fusion transcript

RT-PCR

Gene Amplification in Neuroblastoma

- Neuroblastoma is the most common extracranial solid tumor of childhood.

- These tumors arise in the adrenal medulla and sympathetic ganglia.

- N-*myc* amplification is associated with poor clinical outcome in these cancers.

Gene Amplification in Neuroblastoma
(cont.)

- Tumors with >10 copies of the N-*myc* gene demonstrate poor response to conventional therapy.

- Molecular analysis of these tumors involves differential PCR amplification of the N-*myc* gene and a single-copy reference gene.

Gene Amplification

Tandemly duplicated segment within chromosome/homogeneously staining region (HSR)

Extrachromosomal particles/double minutes

Differential PCR for N-*myc* Gene Amplification

N-myc   GAPDH   N-myc   GAPDH

Co-amplify by PCR and gel electrophoresis

Blank control   Normal control   Non-amplified patient

Blank control   Normal control   Amplified patient

N-myc

GAPDH

Differential PCR for N-*myc* Gene Amplification

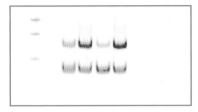

Gene Amplification in Breast Cancer

- Amplification/overexpression of HER2/neu in 25–30% of primary human breast cancers.

- Gene amplification is associated with poor clinical outcome in axillary node positive patients.

- HER2+ patients may benefit from doxorubicin-based adjuvant therapy.

- Patients with HER2+ advanced metastatic breast CA are likely to benefit from Herceptin.

HER2

- Member of growth factor receptor family

- Chromosome 17q21

- 185 kDa transmembrane tyrosine kinase growth factor receptor

- Overexpression due to gene amplification or enhanced transcription

HER2 Detection

- Immunohistochemistry
- dPCR
- FISH

Proteomics specifically addresses Herceptin eligibility, while genomic assays may or may not address this issue. Genomic assays are approved for chemotherapy regimens (adriamycin).

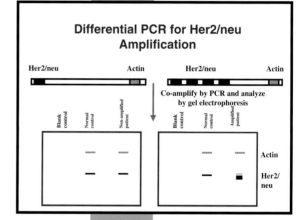

Differential PCR for Her2/neu Amplification

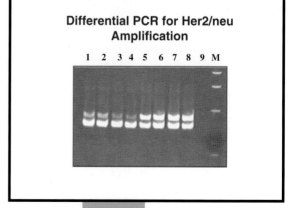

Differential PCR for Her2/neu Amplification

Potential Benefits of Genetic Testing to Cancer Patients

- Cancer risk assessment
- Early detection of tumors
- Specific classification and/or diagnosis of tumor type
- Prognosis (prediction of patient outcome)

Ethical Issues Related to Genetic Testing

- Patient autonomy (right to know or not to know)
- Genetic discrimination
- Confidentiality
- DNA "ownership"

Ethical Issues Related to Genetic Testing *(cont.)*

- Genetic testing in the absence of appropriate therapy or treatment
- Affordability/availability
- Informed consent by patient
- Psychological impact on patient (or family)

SECTION 11

Hematopathology

Goal

To introduce essential concepts in B-cell and T-cell development, immune system diversity related to immunoglobulin gene rearrangements, chromosome rearrangements related to neoplastic transformation, and how these gene rearrangements can be used to determine clonality in lymphoid malignancies using Southern blot or PCR analysis.

Outline

- Classification and diagnosis of lymphoid malignancies
- Determination of clonality
- Southern blot analysis of gene rearrangements
- PCR analysis of gene rearrangements
- Gene rearrangements in non-Hodgkin's lymphoma
- PCR Detection of EBV in Hodgkin's disease

Lymphoid Malignancies

- Acute lymphocytic leukemia
- Chronic lymphoid leukemias
- Non-Hodgkin's lymphomas
- Hodgkin's disease

Real Classification, Blood 1994

Diagnosis of Lymphoma
Multiparameter Approach

- Traditional H&E stained tissue sections (standard of diagnosis)

- Immunopathological methods (routine)

- Molecular genetic methods (common)

- Histochemical stains (select cases)

- Cytogenetic techniques (select cases)

Diagnosis of Lymphoma
Historical

Prior to 1980:   Diagnosis based on morphology

1980:   Introduction of immunopathology

1980's: Rapid growth in immunopathology

1985:   Introduction of molecular genetics

1985 to   Rapid growth in molecular genetic
present: applications

Normal Stages of B-cell Development

	Progenitor B-cell	Pre, Pre B-cell	Pre B-cell	Immature B-cell	Mature B-cell	Activated B-cell	Plasma cell
	TdT	TdT	mu TdT				cIg
IgR:							
Mu							
Kappa							
Lambda							
Surface Ag:							
HLADr							
CD19							
CD20							
CD10							
CD38							
sIg							
Neoplasms	Pre, Pre-B ALL	Pre-B ALL		CLL, B-cell lymphomas			Myeloma

Normal Stages of T-Cell Development

Molecular Genetic Methods

Applications

- Determination of B- and T-cell clonality

Gold Standard
- Determination of B- and T-cell lineage.
- Detection of chromosomal translocations.
  Examples: *bcl*-1 in mantle cell lymphoma
  bcl-2 in follicular lymphoma
- Detection of minimal residual disease
- Detection of viruses (EBV)

B- and T-cell Ontogeny

Theory of lymphoid neoplasia: Disorders of lymphoid cells represent cells arrested at various stages in the normal differentiation scheme.

Surface Immunoglobulin and T-cell Receptors

- Involved in the process of *antigen recognition* by normal B- and T-cells

- **Structurally similar**: Heterodimer proteins linked by disulfide bonds; composed of variable (V) and constant (C) regions

- **Genetically similar**: Consist of a large number of exons ⇨ DNA recombination ⇨ functional receptor

Immune System

- **Diversity:** Must be able to recognize a wide variety of antigens

- **DNA recombination**: Large number of V, D, J and C segments can be transcribed and translated to millions of antigen receptors

- **Somatic mutation**: Allows for even more diversity

Determination of Clonality

- **Definition:** Population of cells with similar characteristics that are all derived from a single precursor cell.

- **Morphology**: Monomorphous cell population

- **Immunopathology**: Monotypic SIg

- **Cytogenetics**: Recurrent chromosomal alteration (e.g., translocation)

- **Molecular genetics**: Clonal B- or T-cell gene rearrangements (Southern blot or PCR)

_____

_____

_____

_____

_____

_____

Southern Blot

- Popular method for determining B- and T-cell clonality

- Uses **DNA probes** (large segments of DNA that recognize primarily J or C segments)

- May detect as little as a 1–5% clonal population

_____

_____

_____

_____

_____

_____

DNA Probes

B Cell
- J_H: Recognizes heavy chain J segments

- J_K: Recognizes kappa light chain J segments

T Cell
- J_{B1B2}: Recognizes J segments in both *B*-chain groups

- CT_B: Recognizes C segments in both *B*-chain groups

_____

_____

_____

_____

_____

Gene Rearrangements

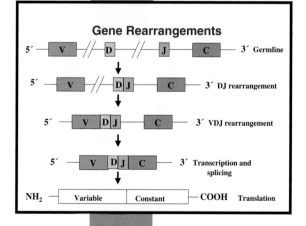

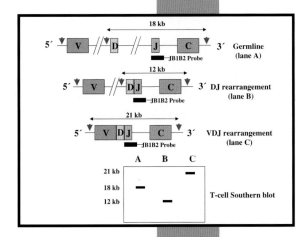

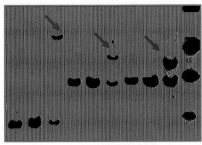

T-cell Southern Blot Analysis for Clonality

1 2 3 4 5 6 7 8 9 M

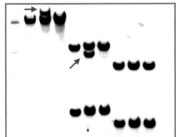

T-cell Southern Blot Analysis for Clonality

M 1 2 3 4 5 6 7 8 9

Southern Blot Interpretation

Clonal rearrangement—*Definition*
- Requires the identification of at least 2 novel bands.
- Novel bands may be present in 2 separate enzyme digests or both present in the same enzyme digest.

Novel band—any band other than
- A germline band
- A cross-hybridization band
- A partial digest band

Polymerase Chain Reaction

- Increasingly popular method to evaluate for the presence of B- or T-cell clonality.
- Analogous to the Southern blot, involves evaluation of segments of DNA that code for the variable regions of the immunoglobulin and T-cell receptor (V and J segments).
- Uses <u>consensus</u> V and J segment primers (recognize shared DNA sequences).
- May detect a 0.1% clonal population.

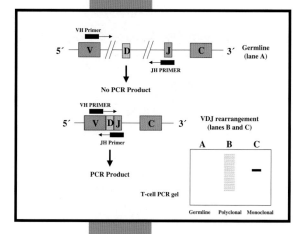

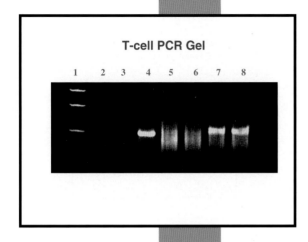

T-cell PCR Gel

1 2 3 4 5 6 7 8

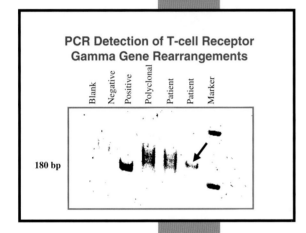

PCR Detection of T-cell Receptor Gamma Gene Rearrangements

Blank
Negative
Positive
Polyclonal
Patient
Patient
Marker

180 bp

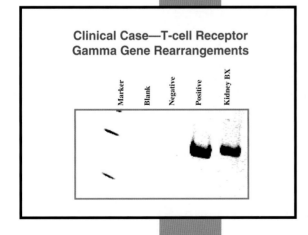

Clinical Case—T-cell Receptor Gamma Gene Rearrangements

Marker
Blank
Negative
Positive
Kidney BX

One year post-kidney biopsy, bone marrow
shows clonal population of T-cells.

Chromosome Translocations in Non-Hodgkin's Lymphoma

- A number of *nonrandom* translocations associated with specific subtypes of non-Hodgkin's lymphoma
- <u>Examples</u>: *bcl*-1 in mantle cell lymphoma
  bcl-2 in follicular lymphoma
- Demonstrable by Southern blot, PCR and FISH
- Identification may help confirm a diagnosis
- Used to monitor patients for evidence of minimal residual disease

Proto-oncogene *bcl*-2

- Normally resides on chromosome 18
- Involved in blocking *apoptosis* (programmed cell death)
- Expression limited to long lived cells
- In FCCL, *bcl*-2 becomes overexpressed following t(14;18) ⟹ extends lifespan of follicular center cells
- Translocation occurs in 80–90% of cases

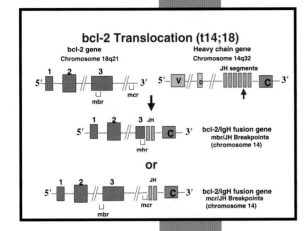

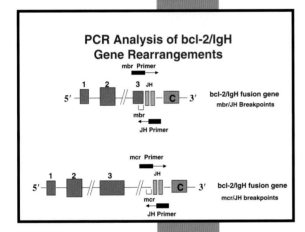

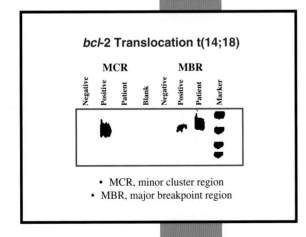

---

bcl-1 Translocation (t11;14)(q13;q32)

MCL-1   MCL-2

Positive | Patient | Patient | Blank | Negative | Positive | Patient | Patient | Marker

---

Hodgkin's Disease

- Diagnosis based on finding neoplastic Reed-Sternberg (RS) cells in a benign inflammatory cell background
- Immunopathological studies confirmatory
- Southern blot and PCR methods not used routinely to establish diagnosis; most cases negative
- Major contribution of molecular genetics has been to elucidate origin of the RS cell

---

Reed-Sternberg Cell

- Cell of origin has been an enigma for decades
- Cells implicated:
  - Histiocytes
  - Interdigitating reticulum cells
  - Dendritic reticulum cells
  - Granulocytes
  - B- and T-lymphocytes
  - Fusions between lymphocytes
  - Fusions between lymphocytes and histiocytes
  - Virally infected cells

Origin of Reed-Sternberg Cell

- Today, the weight of the evidence suggests that the Reed-Sternberg cell is of B-cell or T-cell origin.

- Based on developments in:
  - Immunopathology
  - Microbiology
  - Cell culture methods
  - Molecular genetics

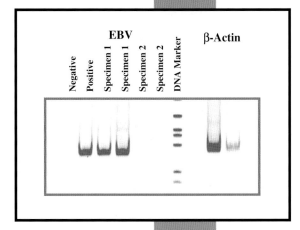

Infectious Disease

Goal

To introduce essential concepts related to the genomes of infectious agents and the application of molecular technologies to the analysis of these agents, including detection of infectious agents, identification of specific agents, molecular strain typing, and monitoring infection and therapy.

Outline

- Applications of molecular analyses to infectious disease
- Molecular diagnosis of EBV
- Molecular diagnosis of parvovirus
- Molecular diagnosis of sexually transmitted diseases
- Human papilloma virus and cervical cancer
- Molecular strain typing and clinical practice
- Molecular analysis of HIV infection
- Hepatitis virus genotyping
- LiPA in infectious disease testing

Applications of Molecular Analyses to Infectious Diseases

- Qualitative detection
- Quantitative detection
- Microbial "identity" testing
- Genotyping/drug resistance

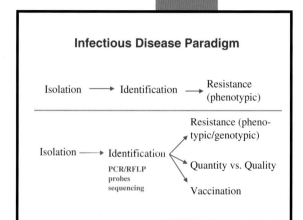

Infectious Disease Paradigm

Isolation ⟶ Identification ⟶ Resistance (phenotypic)

Isolation ⟶ Identification → Resistance (phenotypic/genotypic)
PCR/RFLP → Quantity vs. Quality
probes
sequencing → Vaccination

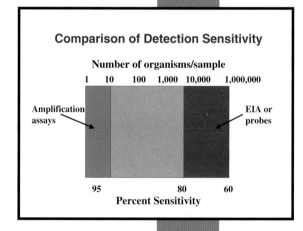

Comparison of Detection Sensitivity

Number of organisms/sample

1   10   100   1,000   10,000   1,000,000

Amplification assays   EIA or probes

95   80   60

Percent Sensitivity

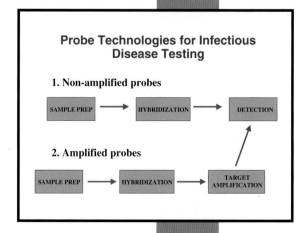

Probe Technologies for Infectious Disease Testing

1. Non-amplified probes

SAMPLE PREP ⟶ HYBRIDIZATION ⟶ DETECTION

2. Amplified probes

SAMPLE PREP ⟶ HYBRIDIZATION ⟶ TARGET AMPLIFICATION

279

_____

_____

_____

_____

_____

_____

_____

_____

_____

_____

_____

_____

_____

_____

_____

_____

_____

_____

_____

Epstein-Barr Virus (EBV)

- Human herpes virus-4 (HHV-4)

- Present in 90% of world population

- Transmission by contact with salivary fluids of active viral shedders ("kissing disease")

- Establishes lifelong latency in B lymphocytes

- Linear dsDNA wrapped around a protein core within a nucleocapsid

Epstein-Barr Virus (EBV)

- **Infectious mononucleosis**
  - Lytic infection in oropharyngeal epithelium
  - Haedache, malaise, chills, cough, nausea, anorexia, myalgia, fever, pharyngitis, lymphadenopathy
- **Burkitt's lymphoma**
  - Most common tumor of childhood in developing countries
  - B-cell lymphoid malignancy
- **Nasopharyngeal carcinoma**
  - Virus present in neoplastic epithelial cells
  - Most often arise near opening of eustachian tube
  - Poor prognosis

EBV in Immunodeficient Patients

- **Posttransplant lymphoproliferative patients**
  - Arise following organ or bone marrow transplant
  - EBV present in 90–95% of cases
- **AIDS patients**
  - 10% of AIDS patients develop lymphoma
  - CNS involvement then 100% contain EBV

Diagnosis of EBV

- Viral culture (3–4 weeks)
- Paul Bunnell (PB) heterophil antibody test (agglutination)
- EBV specific antibodies
  - Immunofluorescence
  - ELISA (enzyme-linked immunosorbent assay) for anti-EBV Abs
- Immunohistochemistry
- Molecular
  - ISH
  - Southern blot
  - PCR (1 EBV genome in 10^6 cells)

Direct Qualitative PCR

EBV Detection

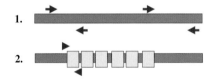

Bam HI-W repetitive region (296 bp) Conserved among EBV Strains

PCR Detection of EBV

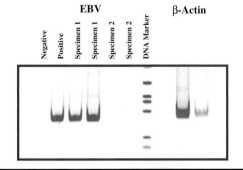

Molecular Diagnosis of EBV

- Direct qualitative detection
- Latent versus active (lytic) infection
  - Terminal repeat elements (0.5 kb sequences)
  - Lytic has linear DNA
  - Latent has closed circular DNA due to joining of repeat ends
  - Repeat elements lost during this change

Molecular Diagnosis of EBV

3.7 kb

4.2 kb **Linear DNA**

(0.5 kb)n

Left = 3.7 kb + 0.5 n kb

Right = 4.2 kb + 0.5 n kb

7.9 kb

Circular DNA

7.9 kb + 0.5n kb

Clonal versus non-clonal??

Parvovirus B19

- Infects only humans
- Very stable, small, round, non-enveloped virus
- 5.6-kb single-stranded DNA molecule
- Transmission through respiratory droplets, across placenta, or from contaminated factor VIII
- Requires actively dividing cells for productive replication
- Infection can be asymptomatic or erythema infectiosum (rash, arthropathy)

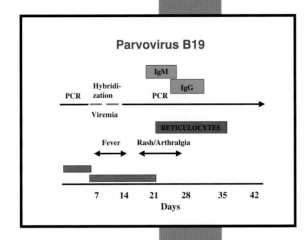

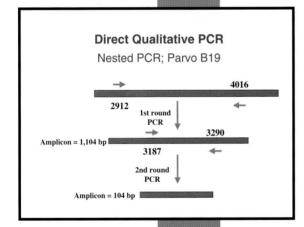

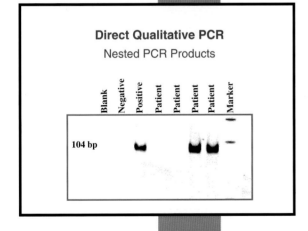

Direct Qualitative PCR Detection

- Single PCR
  - One target sequence
  - Repeated target sequence
- Nested PCR
- PCR followed by probe hybridization

Sexually Transmitted Pathogens

Bacteria	Viruses
• *Chlamydia trachomatis*	• HIV-1 and 2
• *Neisseria gonorrhoeae*	• HTLV-1
• *Treponema pallidum*	• HSV-2
• *Calymmatobacterium granulomatis*	• HPV
• *Ureaplasma urealyticum*	• HBV
	• CMV
	• *Molluscum contagiosum*

Sexually Transmitted Diseases

- 12 million new STD cases/year in the U.S.
- $17 billion overall cost to healthcare
- Can be prevented and/or controlled
  - Behavioral intervention
  - Biomedical intervention

Herpes Simplex Viruses
HSV Types 1 and 2

- Infection occurs worldwide.
- Humans are the only known reservoir.
- Transmission occurs via close contact or sexual activity.
- Most infections are subclinical.
- HSV1 (oral) infection is highest in children <5 years old.
- HSV2 (genital)
  - Females more than males
  - Number of sex partners

HSV Types 1 and 2

- Genital herpes infection increasing in incidence

- Infection is lifelong

  - Painful, recurrent lesions

  - Asymptomatic or sub-clinical infections

  - Rare but serious infections in neonates

HSV Types 1 and 2

- "*herpes*" = to creep
- Oral herpes (HSV1)
  - Acquired in childhood
  - Cold sore, fever blister
  - Reactivation common
- Genital herpes (HSV2)
  - Ulcerative lesions resolve without scarring
  - Extragenital lesions (legs, buttocks)
- Herpes eye infections
  - Unilateral or bilateral conjunctivitis

HSV Types 1 and 2

- Neonatal herpes
  - Potentially fatal
  - High risk of neurological damage
  - Skin, eye, mouth (1/3 of all cases)
  - CNS (50% with neurologic damage)
  - Disseminated infection (multiple organs involved, all with neurologic damage)
- Herpes encephalitis
  - Involves focal areas of temporal lobe
  - If untreated 70% die, few have complete recovery

Pathogenesis of HSV Types 1 and 2

- Infection and replication in epithelial cells of skin or mucosa

- Viral capsids taken up by sensory nerves and transported to neuronal nucleus (latency)

- Virions produced in neuronal nucleus travel down axon to epithelium and produce recurrent disease

HSV Types 1 and 2

- Central core contains dsDNA
- Viral replication
  - Attach to cell membrane
  - Release of capsid into cell
  - VP16 protein escorts viral DNA to cell nucleus
  - Induced transcription of immediate early (alpha) genes
  - These regulate expression of beta genes including DNA polymerase
  - Synthesis of viral DNA and new virions
  - 18- to 20-hour process

Diagnosis of HSV Types 1 and 2

- Culture
- Antigen detection (fluorescent Abs, EIA)
- EM
- Immunohistochemistry
- ISH or Southern blot
- PCR

HSV 1-2 PCR Gel

Turnaround Time

- Viral Isolation
  - Positive result: average 108 hours
  - Negative result: average 154 hours
- PCR
  - Range: 36–72 hours
  - Mean estimated 48 hours

Chlamydia trachomatis
—"The Silent Epidemic"

- Asymptomatic individuals serve as a reservoir of infection.

  - 80% of female infections are asymptomatic

  - 50% of male infections are asymptomatic

Prevalence of *Chlamydia trachomatis*

- Males, 20–24 years

- Females, 15–19 years

- Overall prevalence, 3–5%

- STD clinic populations, >20%

Clinical Syndrome

Males
- Urethritis, epididymitis, proctitis

Females
- Lower genital tract: Cervicitis, urethritis
- Upper genital tract: PID, acute salpingitis
  - Infertility
  - Chronic pelvic pain
  - Ectopic pregnancy

Diagnostic Challenges of
Chlamydia trachomatis Infection

- Misperception of prevalence
- Asymptomatic
- Nonspecific symptoms
- Coinfections
- Unreliable diagnostic tests

_____

_____

_____

_____

_____

_____

Laboratory Diagnosis of
Chlamydia trachomatis Infection

- Culture (gold standard)
- Non-amplified tests
  - Serology
  - EIA
  - Direct fluorescent antibody
  - DNA probe
- *In vitro* amplification tests

_____

_____

_____

_____

_____

LCR and MEIA Detection

Capture Hapten

Detection Hapten

MUP

MU

Unligated probe removed during wash

_____

_____

_____

_____

_____

_____

_____

_____

_____

_____

_____

_____

LCx *Chlamydia trachomatis* Target

- Cryptic plasmid (7–10 copies/organism)
- 48-bp region of the cryptic plasmid
- Unique DNA sequence
- Highly conserved among all *C. trachomatis* serovars
- Contamination control
  - Physical: Closed tube system (no aerosols)
  - Chemical: Inactivation (chelator/oxidizer)

_____

_____

_____

_____

_____

_____

LCx Chlamydia trachomatis

Three-Study Summary

	% Sensitivity	% Specificity
Endocervical	94.4	99.9
Female urine	93.8	99.9
Male urethral	98.0	100.0
Male urine	93.5	99.8
Total	94.6	99.9

_____

_____

_____

_____

_____

_____

Human Papillomavirus (HPV)

Cervical Cancer

- Second most common malignancy in women worldwide

- First solid, malignant tumor recognized as having a viral origin

- 100% preventable by screening for pre-malignant disease

- Highly treatable if detected early

HPV

- Primary cause of cervical cancer.

- Over 70 site-specific types.

- 5–10% of women >35 years of age are persistent carriers of HPV.

- HPV E6 and E7 proteins inhibit p53 and pRB protein functions.

Known Risk Factors for Cervical Cancer

- HPV positivity and specific type
- Persistent HPV infection
- Viral load
- Cytological confirmation of SIL
- Sexual behavior
- Parity
- Epithelial location and characteristics
- Genetic factors

Steps in HPV-induced Cervical Cancer

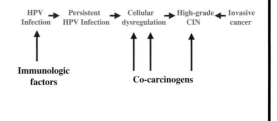

Current Cervical Cancer Screening

The Conventional Pap smear?

- Included in annual GYN examination

- An examination of cervical cells

- Two-thirds reduction in cervical cancer since introduced in the 1950s

- Proven value for mass screening

Limitations of the Conventional Pap Smear

- Does not test for the cause of cervical cancer
- Subjectivity and variability
- Sensitivity and specificity
- Sampling errors
- Interval between Pap tests
- Non-prognostic
- Patient compliance

Bethesda System

- WNL (Within Normal Limits)

  – Includes reactive and reparative changes

- ASCUS (Atypical Squamous Cells of Undetermined Significance)

  – A borderline category of equivocal lesions

Bethesda System *(cont.)*

- LSIL (Low-grade Squamous Intraepithelial Lesions)

  – Combines condylomatous atypia with mild dysplasia (CIN 1)

- HSIL (High-grade Squamous Intraepithelial Lesions)

  – Combines moderate with severe dysplasia (CIN 2 & 3)

- Squamous cell carcinoma

ASCUS Management: The Dilemma

ASCUS diagnosis

Disease present	No disease present
Colposcopy/treatment	Falsely tagged. No colposcopy required.

Past Suggestions for Equivocal Cervical Cytology

- Repeat Pap test (3–6 months)
  - May delay or miss detection of significant disease
  - Patient anxiety while waiting for resolution of first Pap smear
  - Sensitivity of only 76.2%

Past Suggestions for Equivocal Cervical Cytology *(cont.)*

- Colposcopy
  - Up to 78% of ASCUS reports are normal on colposcopy
  - As much as $300–$1200 is added to management costs
  - Patient anxiety over risk of cancer
  - Invasive procedure
  - Largest proportion of HSIL comes from women whose Pap smears are reported ASCUS

Clinical Relevance of Hybrid Capture® II HPV Testing

- 97% Sensitivity: More effective in detecting HSIL than repeat Pap

- Directly detects the underlying cause of cervical cancer

- 99.9% negative predictive value for women with two negative HPV results

Clinical Relevance of
Hybrid Capture® II HPV Testing *(cont.)*

- Helps clarify ambiguous cytology results and identifies persistent infection in women over 35

- Earlier indication of disease, enabling immediate treatment to improve clinical outcomes and reduce patient anxiety

HPV Risk Types

Digene's HPV DNA test uses two RNA probe cocktails to differentiate between carcinogenic and low-risk HPV types.

- Low risk
  - 6, 11, 42, 43, 44
- High risk
  - 16, 18, 31, 33, 35, 39, 45, 51, 52, 56, 58, 59, 68

Prognostic Value of High-risk
Genotype HPV Infection

Prospective studies have shown that 28% of HPV DNA-positive women (cytology normal) developed (SIL) within 2 years compared to only 3% of HPV DNA negative women.

Prognostic Value of Persistent High-risk Type HPV Infection

- 60–70% of women who are HPV positive and cytology negative will develop their first abnormal Pap smear within 4 years.

- HPV detection in women >30 is likely to represent persistent infection.

- The positive predictive value of HPV DNA for the detection of CIN rises with age, whereas that of cytology decreases.

Patient Management Using HPV Triage

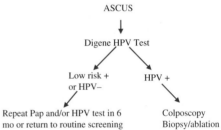

Hybrid Capture® II HPV DNATest Specimen Collection

- Cervical Sampler™ specimen storage and transport
- Cervical samples
  - Storage and shipment up to 2 weeks at 2–30 °C
  - Remaining storage at 2–8 °C for up to 1 week
  - Long-term storage at –20 °C for up to 3 months
- Cervical Biopsies
  - Shipped overnight at 2–30 °C
  - Stored at –20 °C for up to 3 months

Sample Preparation
The ThinPrep® Pap Test™

- Simple change for physician
- Addresses Pap limitations

Digene's Hybrid Capture® II HPV DNATest

- Simple and efficient procedure
- High clinical sensitivity for major carcinogenic HPV types
- High inter- and intra-test reproducibility
- Objective, geographically standardized results
- Simple lab set-up and training
- Amenable to large testing volumes

Release and denature nucleic acids

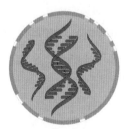

_____

_____

_____

_____

_____

_____

_____

Hybridize RNA probe with target DNA

_____

_____

_____

_____

_____

_____

_____

Capture RNA:DNA hybrids onto a solid phase (in tube or microplate format)

_____

_____

_____

_____

_____

_____

_____

React captured hybrids with multiple antibody conjugates

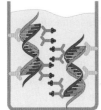

Detect amplified chemiluminescent signal

Increasing Sensitivity/Specificity of PCR

- Target repetitive sequences
- Nested PCR
- PCR + probe hybridization
    - Southern blot
    - Dot blot
    - Liquid hybridization

Strain Typing
Staphylococcus aureus

- Common pathogen responsible for many nosocomial infections

- Main cause of food intoxication

- Increase in methicillin resistant *S. aureus* (MRSA) (mecA gene)

- Identification of toxin genotypes

_____

_____

_____

_____

_____

_____

Strain Typing
Staphylococcus aureus

- Different strains, different extracellular protein toxins
  - Enterotoxin (SEA,SEB,SEC,SED,SEE,SEH)
  - Toxic shock syndrome toxin-1 (TSST-1)
  - Exfoliative toxin (ETA, ETB)
  - Hemolysin
  - Coagulase

_____

_____

_____

_____

_____

_____

Qualitative Detection/Speciation

- Simultaneous detection and speciation
- Conservative vs. unique DNA sequences
- PCR + probe
- PCR + restriction digest
- PCR + sequencing

_____

_____

_____

_____

_____

_____

Mycobacteria

- Increases incidence of tuberculosis, among other diseases.
- Multiple co-infections reported in immunocompromised hosts
- Treatment dependent upon species identified (TB vs. others)
- Identification taking up to several months
- Some Mycobacteria (i.e. *M. leprae*) cannot be cultured

Mycobacteria

- HIV impact on tuberculosis
- *M. avium – M. intracellulare* (MAI) complex associated with immunosuppression
- Opportunistic Mycobacteria
  - *M. kansasii*
  - *M. xenopi*
  - *M. fortuitum*
  - *M. scrofulaceum*

Mycobacteria

- DNA coding for 16S subunit of rRNA
  - Unique sequence to all Mycobacteria
  - Single copy
  - Probe hybridization to speciate
- Insertion sequence 6110 (IS6110)
  - Specific for *M. tuberculosis*
  - Multiple copies

Mycobacteria

- hsp65 gene present in all Mycobacteria
- Restriction digest with BstEII and HaeIII

	BstEII	HaeIII
M. tuberculosis	245/120/80	160/140/70
M. avium	245/220	140/105
M. genavense	325/120	140/105

Mycobacteria

- *M. tuberculosis* genes rpoB and katG
- Mutations predict resistance to rifampin and isoniazid
- Microbial relatedness
  - Identify outbreaks of infection
  - Determine mode of acquisition of a pathogen
  - Analyze individual patients (determine if relapse or different infection)
  - Define effective preventive and therapeutic measures

Nosocomial Infection

- \>2 million cases per year
- \>$5.0 billion in healthcare costs
- Molecular epidemiology/infection control
- Molecular strain typing (pulsed field gel electrophoresis)

Molecular Strain Typing and Clinical Practice

- Investigation of the spread of drug-resistant pathogens
- Evaluation of multiple isolates from the same patient
- Differentiation of relapse from new infection
- Epidemiology/infection control

Pulse Field Gel Electrophoresis

- Culture
- Embed pellet in agarose plug
- Treat with cell lysis (lysozyme)
- Proteinase K treatment
- Restriction enzyme digestion
- Gel electrophoresis

Pulse Field Gel Electrophoresis
Interpretation

- Class I: Identical (band patterns are the same)
- Class II: Closely related (differ by one genetic event [1–3 band difference]; samples are subtypes)
- Class III: Possibly related (differ by 2 genetic events [4–5 band difference]; may be subtypes)
- Class IV: Different (differ by >3 genetic events [>6 band difference]; different strains)

Molecular Strain Typing
Staphylococcus aureus

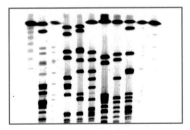

HIV Viral Load

- Not a diagnostic assay
- Does not replace CD4 counts
  - Initiation of anti-retroviral therapy
  - Prophylaxis for opportunistic infections
- Predicts slow or rapid progression to AIDS
- Monitoring response to anti-retroviral therapy

Recommended Frequency for HIV Viral Load Testing

- Two baseline measurements (2–4 weeks apart, not within 1 month of acute illness or vaccination)
- 3–4 weeks after changing or initiating therapy
- Every 3–4 months with CD4 counts to determine if the response to therapy is persisting

Molecular Laboratory Methods for Quantitating HIV-1 RNA

- AMPLICOR HIV monitor (RT-PCR)
- Branched DNA assay (bDNA)
- Nucleic acid sequence-based amplification (NASBA)

HIV Viral Load Methodology Comparison

	AMPLICOR	bDNA	NASBA
Specimen requirement	EDTA	EDTA	Any anticoag.
Volume of plasma	200 mL	1 mL	100 mL–1 mL
Sensitivity (copies/ml)	400 (50)	100	400
FDA approval	YES	NO	NO

HIV-1 Lifecycle

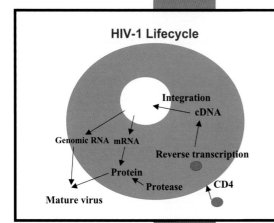

Integration

cDNA

Genomic RNA mRNA

Reverse transcription

Protein

Protease

CD4

Mature virus

HIV Treatment Options

Nucleoside <u>reverse transcriptase</u> inhibitors

- Zidovudine (AZT)(Retrovir)
  - Didanosine (Videx)
  - Zalcitabine (Hivid)
  - Lamivudine (Epivir)
  - Stavudine (Zerit)

(M41L, M184V, L210W,T215Y)

_____

_____

_____

_____

_____

_____

_____

_____

_____

_____

_____

_____

_____

_____

_____

_____

_____

_____

HIV Treatment Options *(cont.)*

Protease inhibitors

- Saquinavir (Invirase)
- Nelfinavir (Viracept)
- Indinavir (Crixivan)
- Ritonavir (Norvir)

(L10I, M46L, G48V, I54A, L63T, I64V,V77I,V82A)

HIV Viral Load as Predictor of Time to the Onset of AIDS

Viral load (copies/mL)	Time to onset (years)
<500	>10
500–3,000	>10
3,000–10,000	8.3
10,000–30,000	5.8
>30,000	2.8

Guidelines for Using HIV Viral Load Assays In Clinical Practice

• Plasma HIV RNA level that suggests initiation of treatment	>5,000–10,000 copies and CD4 count suggestive of progression or >30,000–50,000 copies
• Target level of HIV RNA after initiation of treatment	Undetectable; <5,000 copies
• Minimal decrease in HIV RNA indicative of antiviral activity	>0.5 log decrease (3-fold)
• Change in HIV RNA level that suggests treatment failure	Return to pre-treatment value or within 0.3 – 0.5 log

Saag *et al., Nature Medicine* 1996;2:625–629.

Viral Genotyping

All viruses have demonstrated
the potential to generate
sequence diversity.

Types of Sequence Diversity

- Natural (HCV subtypes, HPV
  strains)

- Drug selected/induced resistance

Viral Sequence Diversity

Replication = Resistance

Hepatitis

- Acute and chronic

- Acute is self-limiting and complete recovery

- Some acute cases become chronic

Hepatitis *(cont.)*

- 80–90% caused by acute viral infection with hepatitis A (HAV), B (HBV), or C (HCV) virus

- 5–10% due to alcohol consumption

- <5% due to autoimmune disease or metabolic disorders (Wilson's disease)

Hepatitis A

- Most common cause of hepatitis in children

- Spread by fecal-oral route (poor sanitation, contaminated food)

- Short incubation period

- Complete recovery

- RNA virus

Hepatitis B

- Most common form of hepatitis worldwide

- Decreased incidence due to hepatitis B vaccine

- Spread by sex, serum, mother to baby

- Circular dsDNA virus

_____

_____

_____

_____

_____

_____

Hepatitis C

- Post-transfusion hepatitis

- Majority of infections become chronic

- Spread by serum, sex, and/or other

- RNA virus

- HCV RNA is first marker to appear with acute infection (1–2 weeks)

_____

_____

_____

_____

_____

_____

Chronic Hepatitis

- Ongoing damage to liver

- Most patients asymptomatic

- Development of cirrhosis and/or hepatocellular carcinoma

- Most commonly due to HCV or HBV

_____

_____

_____

_____

_____

_____

_____

_____

_____

_____

_____

_____

_____

_____

_____

_____

_____

_____

_____

_____

_____

_____

_____

_____

_____

_____

| **HCV Infection Morbidity and Mortality** |
| United States, 1995 |

• Newly acquired infections	28,000
• Newly acquired symptomatic	8,400
• Deaths from fulminant hepatic failure	Rare
• Prevalence rate of anti-HCV	1.8%
• Chronic infections	3.9 million
• Deaths from chronic disease	8,000–10,000

HCV Genome

- Single-stranded RNA genome

- 9,400 bp

- High mutation rate

- Exists as a population of slightly different viruses quasispecies)

HCV Genome

Structural   Nonstructural

C	E1	E2	NS2	NS3	NS4	NS5

Core   Envelope   Protease   RNA POL

HCV Genotypes

- Six major groups or genotypes

- Numerous subtypes

- Homology between viruses of different types: <69%

- Homology between viruses of the same type: approximately 79%

- Homology between viruses of same subtype: >88%

- Genotypes differ in geographic distribution

Clinical Utility of HCV Genotyping

- Epidemiology

- Severity of disease

- Rate of disease progression (i.e., TX pts with type 1B)

- Impact on diagnostic assays

- Response to therapy

Interferon α 2b Plus Ribavirin for Initial Therapy of Chronic HCV

	Sustained Virologic Response	
Genotype	24 weeks	48 weeks
1,4,5,or 6	32/177 (18%)	56/180 (31%)
2 or 3	64/100 (64%)	62/97 (64%)

Poynard et al. Lancet 1998;326:142.

_____

_____

_____

_____

_____

_____

_____

What is LiPA?

- LiPA is a **Li**ne **P**robe **A**ssay (INNOGENETICS).

- Reverse hybridization assay using sequence-specific oligonucleotide probes (reverse SSOP)

- Provides multi-parameter testing in a single-strip format

_____

_____

_____

_____

_____

_____

LiPA —
Step 1. Nucleic Acid Isolation

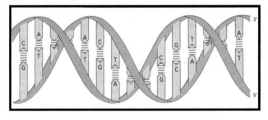

_____

_____

_____

_____

_____

Lipa–
Step 2. Amplification

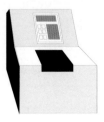

Isolation and Amplification for
the INNO-LiPA HCV II Assay

- Standard assay uses 50 μl of serum.
- Isolate HCV RNA by treatment with guanidinium/phenol (TRIzol LS).
- Precipitate and perform cDNA synthesis with random priming and AMV-RT.
- Perform first-round amplification.
- Perform gel analysis with Gel Control.
- Perform second round amplification. (Only if first-round amplification control is insufficient)

LiPA —
Step 3. Hybridization

ssDNA

Trough →

INNO-LiPA HCV II

Principles of the Technique

- Denaturation of amplified product.
- Reverse hybridization to 21 type and subtype specific probes.
- Conjugate and amplification controls on nitocellulose strip.
- Steptavidin labeled with alkaline phosphatase is added and binds to any biotinylated hybrid previously formed.
- Incubation with substrates BCIP (5-bromo-4-chloro-3-indolyl phosphate and NBT (nitro blue tetrazolium) results in a purple precipitate.
- Read genotype using interpretation chart.

LiPA —
Step 4. Stringent Wash

Biotinylated amplicon

Sequence-specific oligonucleotide probes

LiPA —
Step 5. Conjugate Incubation

Biotinylated amplicon

Type and Subtype-Specific Probe Location on the INNO-LiPA HCV II Strip

Oligonucleotide probes were designed to cover 7 variable regions within the 5´ NTR using the HCV nucleotide sequence database at the National Center for Biotechnology Information (n = 448 as of 12/95).

Probes were selected by consideration of nucleotide composition (%G+C), length, target strand (sense or anti-sense), and hybridization temperature.

TYPE   SUBTYPE

Marker line
Conjugate control
Amplification control
1
1a
1b
1b
1a/1b
2
2a/2c
2b
3
4
5a
6a

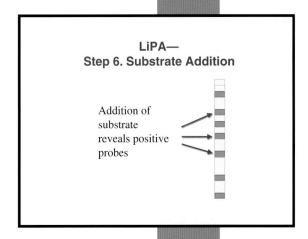

LiPA—
Step 6. Substrate Addition

Addition of
substrate
reveals positive
probes

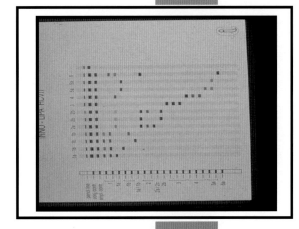

Identity Testing

_____

_____

_____

_____

_____

_____

_____

_____

_____

_____

_____

_____

_____

_____

_____

_____

_____

_____

_____

_____

Goal

To introduce essential concepts in identity testing through molecular analysis of DNA, and to describe examples of applications of identity testing for the clinical laboratory, including case studies.

Outline

- Historical developments in identity testing
- DNA-based identity testing
- The first cases using DNA-based identity testing
- PCR analysis of STRs
- Parentage testing
- Applications of identity testing in the clinical laboratory
- Bone marrow transplant engraftment analysis
- Clinical case studies

Identity Testing and Forensic DNA Analysis

- Criminalistic investigation

- Immigration

- Parentage

- Clinical

Identity Testing

1800s	Fingerprint
1900	ABO blood group typing
1960s	HLA typing
1980s	DNA analysis (VNTRs)
1990s	DNA analysis (STRs)

The First Case, 1985

A young boy from Ghana leaves the U.K. to be reunited with his father in Ghana. He then returns to the U.K. to be reunited with his mother.

Was he the son or the nephew of this woman?

HLA techniques at that time were too crude to resolve this issue. Using minisatellite probes for hypervariable regions in human DNA, Alec Jeffreys indisputably showed that this was indeed the son and not the nephew of this woman. This immigration case led the way for DNA fingerprinting.

The First Murder Case, 1986

Two schoolgirls in the quiet town of Leicester were murdered, one in 1983 and one in 1986. The circumstances of the rapes and murder were identical. So when a young man confessed, the authorities thought they had the assailant for both crimes. Semen swabs had been taken from both girls and DNA analysis was requested. The samples were from the same individual, but not the one who had confessed.

The First Murder Case, 1986 *(cont.)*

A call was then put out to all local males between the ages of 17 and 34 to be subjected to DNA fingerprint analysis. The true murderer had a workmate go in his place. As the investigation dragged on, the proxy told a friend at the local pub that he had stood in for someone as part of the DNA test. A woman overheard the conversation and reported this to authorities.

DNA-based Identity Testing

- DNA, the molecular basis of heredity
- DNA, a very polymorphic molecule
- VNTR = variable number of tandem repeats (14–30 bp)
- STR = short tandem repeats (di-, tri-, tetranucleotide repeats)
- DNA sequence polymorphism = one base difference

Polymorphic Allelic Variation in DNA

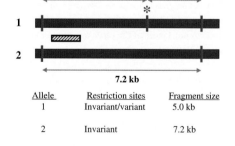

Allele	Restriction sites	Fragment size
1	Invariant/variant	5.0 kb
2	Invariant	7.2 kb

Variable Number of Tandem Repeat Polymorphisms

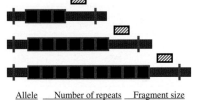

Allele	Number of repeats	Fragment size
1	3	200 bp
2	6	230 bp
3	9	260 bp

PCR Analysis of STRs

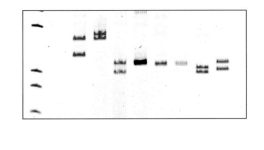

Reverse Dot Blot Analysis Using Antisense Oligonucleotide Probes

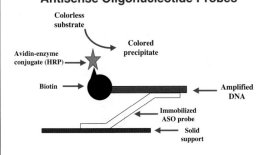

**Reverse Dot Blot Analysis Using
Antisense Oligonucleotide Probes**

**PM+DQA1 Amplification
and Typing Kit**

- HLA DQA1 (6)
- Low-density lipoprotein receptor (LDLR) (2)
- Glycophorin A (GYPA) (2)
- Hemoglobin G gamma globulin (HBGG) (3)
- D7S8 (2)
- Group-specific component (GC) (3)

PM PCR Amplification and Typing Kit
Power of Discrimination

- PM ONLY:
  - African American (0.9949)
  - U.S. Caucasian (0.9953)
  - U.S. Hispanic (0.9962)
- PM + HLA DQA1:
  - African American (0.9997)
  - U.S. Caucasian (0.9998)
  - U.S. Hispanic (0.9998)

DNA-based Parentage Testing
Mendelian Principles

- **Law of Segregation**
  - Each gamete carries only one allele for a gene.
  - Each allele is equally represented.

- **Law of Independent Assortment**
  - The segregation of alleles of one gene are independent of the segregation of the alleles of another gene.

Genotype Frequency in Diallelic System

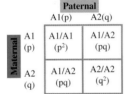

		Paternal	
		A1(p)	A2(q)
Maternal	A1 (p)	A1/A1 (p^2)	A1/A2 (pq)
	A2 (q)	A1/A2 (pq)	A2/A2 (q^2)

p,q = proportion of A1 and A2 alleles in population (p + q = 1)
p^2 = proportion of A1 homozygotes
q^2 = proportion of A2 homozygotes
2pq = proportion of heterozygotes
$p^2 + 2pq + q^2 = 1$

DNA-based Parentage Testing

- Population genetics
  - Various alleles occur with different frequencies depending on racial/ethnic origins of subjects.
- Useful polymorphic locus must
  - have a high degree of heterozygosity.
  - have a low rate of recombination.
  - confer no selective advantage.
  - be inherited codominantly.

DNA-based Parentage Testing

- Collect specimens with chain of custody
- Extract DNA, perform analysis
- Size resultant bands at each locus
- Determine allele frequencies
- Calculate
  - PI (paternity index)
  - CPI (cumulative paternity index)
  - CPP (cumulative probability of paternity)
- Issue report

Parentage Testing

Participants

- Mother (not absolutely required)

- Child

- Alleged father (accused or suspected of being biological father; testing biased in his favor; must achieve a cumulative probability of paternity of >99%)

Chain of Custody

- Verify identity of subject providing specimen; include photographs

- Document each step of handling, transport, and processing of specimen

- Store specimen in secure environment

Parentage Testing

Bayesian Analysis of Paternity

- X = factors favoring paternity, gamete frequency (0, 0.5, OR 1) (normal, heterozygous, homozygous)

- Y = factors against paternity, allele frequency in appropriate population

- PI = paternity index (X/Y); likelihood that matching allele is a result of alleged father being the biological father

DNA-based Parentage Testing

- PI/(PI+1) $\times$ 100 = probability of paternity (derived from Bayesian analysis)

- Cumulative probability of paternity (CPP): Multiply paternity index for each locus tested to calculate cumulative paternity index (CPI)

- CPI = $(PI_A \times PI_B \times PI_C \ldots)$

- CPP = (CPI/CPI + 1) $\times$ 100

DNA-based Parentage Testing

- **Exclusion**: When an alleged father does not share the obligate paternal allele with the child at two or more loci

- **Non-exclusion**: When an alleged father shares all obligate paternal alleles with the child

DNA-based Parentage Testing Case Results

System	Mother	Child	Alleged Father	Paternity Index
D3S1358	17,18	17,18	17,18	2.72
VWA	15,17	15,19	18,19	4.55
D16S539	12,13	12	11,12	1.46
D2S1338	24	20,24	20,23	3.70
D8S1179	13,14	13,14	11,14	2.00
D21S11	31.2,32.2	31.2,32	31.2,32	40.00
D18S51	12,15	11,12	11,17	25.00
D19S433	14,15	14,15	14,16	1.32
THO1	9.3	9,9.3	9,9.3	3.64
FGA	22,23	23	21,23	3.57

DNA System: Perkin Elmer SGM Plus

CPI: 2,293,551
CPP (prior probability 50%): 99.99%
CPP (prior probability 10%): 99.99%

Conclusion: The alleged father is in all likelihood the biological father of the child.

DNA-based Parentage Testing Case Results

System	Mother	Child	Alleged Father	Paternity Index
D3S1358	16,18	16,17	14,18	—
VWA	18	16,18	17	—
D16S539	11	11,13	11,12	—
D2S1338	17,25	25,26	17,23	—
D8S1179	13,14	13,14	13,15	0.93
D21S11	27,31	27,30	29	—
D19S433	13,15	15,17.2	12,14	—
THO1	6,9	8,9	9.3	—
FGA	18,19	18,22	21,25	—

DNA System: Perkin Elmer SGM Plus

CPI: —
CPP (prior probability 50%): —
CPP (prior probability 10%): —
CPP (prior probability 90%): —

Conclusion: The alleged father can be excluded as the biological father of the child.

Likelihood Ratios (PI)

Child	Mother	AF	PI
q	pq	q	1/q
q	p	q	impossible
pq	p or pr	q	1/q
q	q	q	1/q
pq	p or pr	qr	1/2q
q	p	qr	impossible
q	pq	qr	1/2q
q	q	qr	1/2q
pq	pq	pq	1/(p + q)
pq	pq	q	1/(p + q)
pq	pq	qr	1/(2p + 2q)

Parentage Calculation

System	Mother	Child	AF	PI
DQA1	2,3	2	2,4.1	—
	pq	q	qr	1/2q

Frequency of "2" allele in Caucasians is 0.145
$$1/(2)(0.145) = 1/.29 = 3.45$$

D3S1358	16,17	16,17	16,17	—
	pq	pq	pq	1/(p + q)

Frequencies of 16 and 17 are 0.132 and 0.002
$$1/(0.132 + 0.002) = 1/0.134 = 7.46$$

Parentage Calculation

System	Mother	Child	AF	PI
DQA1	2,3	2	2,4.1	3.45
D3S1358	16,17	16,17	16,17	7.46

$$\text{CPI} = (\text{PIa} \times \text{Pib} \times \ldots)$$
$$\text{CPI} = 3.45 \times 7.46 = 25.74$$

$$\text{CPP} = (\text{CPI/CPI} + 1) \times 100$$
$$\text{CPP} = (25.74/26.74) \times 100 = 96.26\%$$

Applications for Identity Testing in the Clinical Laboratory

- Specimen identification
- Urine donor identification (toxicology)
- Pre-employment drug testing
- Confirmation for other civil cases
- Monitoring bone marrow transplant chimerism

Bone Marrow Transplant Engraftment Analysis

Marker	Female Donor	Male Recipient			
		Buccal	1st	2nd	3rd
LDLR	AA	AB	AB	AB	AA
GYPA	AB	BB	BB(A)	BB(A)	AB
HBGG	AB	AB	AB	AB	AB
D7S8	AB	AB	AB	AB	AB
GC	AC	AC	AC	AC	AC
Y1	Neg	Pos	ND	ND	Neg
N1	Neg	Pos	ND	ND	Neg

Bone Marrow Transplant Engraftment Analysis

Mixed Chimerism

Chimerism (%)	Donor DNA (ng)	Recipient DNA (ng)
0	0	200
1	2	198
2	4	196
5	10	190
10	20	180
25	50	150
50	100	100
75	150	50
90	180	20
95	190	10
98	196	4
99	198	2
100	200	0

Surgical Specimens and Identity Testing

A 41-year-old female had a right breast excisional biopsy performed. At the first post-operative visit she reviewed the pathology report with a surgeon who had not performed the biopsy. The original report indicated that the breast biopsy had been taken from the left breast. Moreover, the surgeon indicated that the dimensions of the biopsy as indicated in the report were inconsistent with the small size of the patient's breast. Review of the accession form indicated that the surgeon had incorrectly indicated the left breast as the site of biopsy.

Surgical Specimens and Identity Testing
(cont.)

The patient's chart and operative note verified a
right-side biopsy. The medical records, reports, and
slides of all three operative breast biopsies performed
on the same day were reviewed. All of the quality
control numbers were concordant, indicating that the
operating room specimens from that day were valid.
Because of the surgeon's insistence that the specimen
size and site were inconsistent, a specimen mix-up
was considered.

Surgical Specimens and Identity Testing

Speciman	DQA1	LDLR	GYPA	HBGG	D7S8	GC
Blank	—	—	—	—	—	—
Kit control	1.1,4	B,B	A,B	A,A	A,B	B,B
Volunteer	4,4	A,A	A,B	A,B	A,B	A,C
S94	2,3	B,B	B,B	A,A	A,A	A,C
S95	2,3	B,B	B,B	A,A	A,A	A,C
Blood	2,3	B,B	B,B	A,A	A,A	A,C

1 in 37,566 Caucasian females

Discrimination Power of PM-DQA1 Testing

Case number	Urine		Blood		Typing	
	260 nm	260/280	260 nm	260/280	DQA1	PM
95-56 (female)	0.186	0.246	0.151	1.987	1.1, 2	AA,AB,AC,AA,BC
95-57 (female)	0.149	0.330	0.113	2.093	3, 3	AA,AB,AA,AB,AA
95-58 (female)	0.106	0.338	0.498	1.894	1.3, 1.2	AA,AA,AB,AA,CC
95-59 (female)	0	—	0.443	1.909	1.1, 1.1	BB,AB,AB,AA,AB
95-60 (female)	0	—	0.145	2.042	1.1, 3	AB,AA,AB,AB,AC
95-61 (male)	0.232	0.396	0.246	1.875	1.2, 1.2	AB,AB,AB,AA,AC

_____

_____

_____

_____

_____

_____

_____

_____

_____

_____

_____

_____

_____

_____

_____

_____

_____

_____

_____

Clinical Case 1

A 51-year-old man underwent core biopsy of the prostate to rule out carcinoma. Several H&E slides were received that showed a fragment of carcinomatous epithelium adjacent to benign prostate core samples. The origin of the neoplastic tissue was questioned.

Sampling of Tissue for DNA Analysis

Apply pinpoint solution to selected tissue area.

Lift off and transfer tissue fragment to tube.

DNA can be further purified on a spin column or used for PCR.

Clinical Case 1
Testing Results

Specimen	LDLR	GYPA	HBGG	D7S8	GC	TPO	THO
Blank	—	—	—	—	—	—	—
Control	B,B	A,B	A,A	A,B	B,B	182/194	243
Prostate	B,B	A,B	A,B	A,A	C,C	230 bp	181 bp
? Tissue	A,B	A,B	A,B	A,A	A,C	230 bp	181/189 bp

Clinical Case 2

A clinical chemistry laboratory performs more than 100,000 tests per month. On one occasion, blood was drawn from patient X several times a day for 8 consecutive days. Routine testing indicated a constant increase in BUN and creatinine. On day 8 a blood specimen was received labeled with the same patient demographics as a previous specimen from one hour earlier. A significant decrease in these two analytes was observed and the labeling questioned.

Clinical Case 2
Analyte Testing Results

Test	Result (patient X)	Result (?)
NA (mmol/L)	135	137
K (mmol/L)	5.0	3.4
CL (mmol/L)	102	109
CO_2 (mmol/L)	20	20
BUN (mg/dL)	102	3
CREAT (mg/dL)	2.5	0.5

Clinical Case 2
DNA Testing Results

Specimen	THO	TPO	CSF	VWA	D7S460	ACTBP2
Blank	—	—	—	—	—	—
Patient X	182/186	231	299/307	134/138	173/177	241
? Blood	186/196	243	315	142/154	178	274/282

_____

_____

_____

_____

_____

_____

_____

_____

_____

_____

_____

_____

_____

Clinical Case 3

A pre-placement urine drug test conducted in a young man was positive for 480 ng/mL benzoylecognine. When contacted by the medical review officer, the donor denied using drugs and said the collector must have mixed up samples.

Clinical Case 3

DNA Testing Results

Specimen	DQA1	LDLR	GYPA	HBGG	D7S8	GC
Blank	—	—	—	—	—	—
Control	1.1,4	B,B	A,B	A,A	A,B	B,B
Urine	1.1,1.2	A,A	A,B	B,B	A,A	B,B
Blood	1.1,1.2	A,A	A,B	B,B	A,A	B,B

Self-assessment
Questions and Answers

Questions

1. Molecular diagnostics utilizes principles of molecular biology to do all of the following except:
   a. identify individuals at risk for acquiring disease
   b. diagnose infectious disease
   c. determine appropriate treatment
   d. increase morbidity

2. In 1953, Watson and Crick described:
   a. the RNA tertiary structure
   b. the DNA double helix
   c. the laws of heredity
   d. a polymerase chain reaction

3. The human genome consists of:
   a. a haploid copy number
   b. 22 chromosomes
   c. a circular structure
   d. approximately 6 billion bases

4. Euchromatin is:
   a. densely packed in the centromeric region of a chromosome
   b. a portion of the mitochondrial genome
   c. a transcribed region of genomic DNA
   d. located in the nucleolus

5. All are true of DNA except:
   a. it is composed or repeating nucleotide subunits
   b. the order of nucleotides represents all of the genetic information in a cell
   c. the sugar moiety is ribose
   d. the structure is a double helix consisting of two polynucleotide strands

Match the following terms by placing the letter from the second column next to the term in the first column.

6. pyrimidne _____   a. adenine

7. purine _____   b. pentose sugar

8. RNA _____   c. G:C

9. nucleoside _____   d. six-member ring

10. three hydrogen bonds _____   e. uracil

11. DNA found in the mitochondria comes from:
    a. intronic nuclear DNA sequences
    b. maternal inheritance
    c. the Golgi complex
    d. viral infection

12. DNA can be denatured by all of the following except:
    a. acidic pH
    b. increased temperature
    c. H-bond solvents
    d. NaOH

13. The central dogma of molecular biology with respect to genetic information is best depicted by:
    a. DNA → transcription → protein → RNA → DNA
    b. DNA → translation → RNA → transcription → DNA
    c. DNA → transcription → RNA → translation → protein
    d. RNA → transcription → DNA → translation → protein

14. A nucleotide is composed of all of the following except:
    a. a phosphate group
    b. phosphodiester bonds
    c. pentose sugar
    d. cyclic nitrogen compound or base

15. An abnormal change in a gene sequence is known as a:
    a. variant
    b. mutation
    c. genotype
    d. segregated allele

16. Purines are double-ring structures and include:
    a. adenine and guanine
    b. cytosine and thymine
    c. adenine and thymine
    d. cytosine and guanine

17. The two strands of DNA that compose the double helix are held together by:
    a. sulfhydroyl bonds
    b. hydrogen bonds
    c. phosphodiester and carbon bonds
    d. nitrogen and hydrogen bonds

18. All of the following contribute to the complementary nature of the two DNA strands except:
   a. the parallel nature of strands
   b. a 5′-3′ and 3′-5′orientation
   c. A:T; G:C
   d. opposite chemical polarity

19. Genomic DNA in a diploid normal human cell is dispersed into:
   a. 23 chromosomes
   b. 46 chromosomes
   c. 69 chromatids
   d. 46 pairs of chromosomes

20. The actual cause of a human disease is known as:
   a. pathogenesis
   b. etiology
   c. clinical phenotype
   d. molecular mechanism

21. Which of the following are E.L.S.I. concerns of the human genome project?
   a. confidentiality
   b. reproductive issues
   c. stigmatization
   d. all of the above

22. In handling clinical specimens, you should always assume:
   a. the specimen is contaminated with ammonium persulfate
   b. the specimen contains infectious agents
   c. the outside of the container is clean
   d. none of the above

23. How much whole blood is typically needed for Southern blot analysis?
   a. 0.5 mL
   b. 1 mL
   c. 5 mL
   d. 0.5 µL

24. Which anticoagulant is not acceptable for molecular analysis?
   a. EDTA
   b. Heparin
   c. ACD
   d. the one found in lavender top blood tubes

25. The recommended storage temperature for bone marrow specimens is:
   a. 22 °C
   b. 25 °C
   c. 4 °C
   d. –20 °C

26. Blood or bone marrow specimens should be:
   a. frozen immediately upon arrival to the lab
   b. treated to lyse RBCs
   c. stored at –20 °C if RNA is needed
   d. none of the above

27. All of the following should be included in the packaging of a specimen for shipment except:
    a. absorbent material
    b. sealed container
    c. paper bag
    d. styrofaom box

28. Cultured cells are shipped:
    a. as dried cell pellets
    b. in flasks full of media
    c. on dry ice
    d. as a non-biohazard material

29. All of the following must be included on a specimen label except:
    a. date of birth
    b. name
    c. social security number
    d. date and time of collection

30. Long -term storage of DNA should be at which temperature?
    a. 4 °C
    b. 20 °C
    c. –20 °C
    d. –70 °C

31. All of the following are steps in DNA isolation except:
    a. protein digestion
    b. cell lysis
    c. precipitation
    d. amplification

32. Organic DNA extraction involves:
    a. phenol
    b. salt precipitation
    c. silica matrices
    d. magnetic beads

33. Quantitating DNA concentration can be performed by:
    a. infrared spectrophotometry
    b. UV spectrophotometry
    c. polyacrylamide gel electrophoresis
    d. all of the above

34. Spectrophotometry is a useful method to analyze nucleic acids because of:
    a. light absorbance
    b. light scatter
    c. light penetration
    d. none of the above

35. Spectrophotometry can provide all of the following data except:
    a. quantity of DNA
    b. quantity of RNA
    c. quality of nucleic acid
    d. purity of nucleic acid

36. Which of the following spectrophotometry readings will yield more DNA?
    a. OD260 = 0.133
    b. OD280 = 0.245
    c. OD260 = 0.022
    d. 260/280 = 1.800

37. You have been given a 1-mm cube of fresh tissue from which to extract DNA. After extracting the entire specimen, you resuspend the DNA in 50 μL of buffer. Using 10 μL in 990 μL buffer for spectrophotometry, the A260 = 0.5 and the A280 = 0.28. The concentration of DNA is:
    a. 2.5 μg/uL
    b. 5 μg/uL
    c. 25 μg/uL
    d. none of the above

38. The 260/280 ratio in the above case indicates:
    a. poor quality
    b. unacceptable purity
    c. acceptable purity
    d. high quality

39. Nucleic acid-modifying enzymes include all of the following except:
    a. restriction endonucleases
    b. polymerases
    c. cyclins
    d. ligases

Match the following terms by placing the letter from the second column next to the term in the first column.

40. allele   ——   a. purine:pyrimidine

41. complementarity ——   b. heterozygous

42. haploid   ——   c. diabetes

43. polygenic   ——   d. promoter

44. transcription   ——   e. sperm cell

45. Restriction endonucleases are characterized by all of the following except:
    a. occuring only in microorganisms
    b. functioning as homodimers
    c. recognizing sequences of 10–15 bp in length
    d. cleaving phosphodiester bonds

46. In setting up a restriction digest, how much enzyme should you use per μg of DNA?
    a. 1 unit
    b. 5 units
    c. 10 units
    d. none of the above

47. All of the following are components of a restriction digest except:
    a. genomic DNA
    b. restriction enzyme
    c. $MgCl_2$
    d. buffer

48. DNA has what net charge?
    a. neutral
    b. positive
    c. negative
    d. none of the above

49. The most suitable whole blood anticoagulant for extraction of nucleic acids is:
    a. EDTA
    b. heparin
    c. iodoacetate
    d. oxalate

50. Contamination of a DNA sample with either protein or phenol will result in:
    a. increase in OD_{260}/OD_{280}
    b. increase in OD_{280}
    c. decrease in OD_{260}
    d. $OD_{260}/OD_{280} = 1.8$

51. The migration rate of a macromolecule through a gel matrix during electrophoresis depends on:
    a. the net charge on the molecule
    b. the size of the molecule
    c. a specific gel matrix
    d. all of the above

52. Agarose and polyacrylamide gel matrices differ with respect to:
    a. gel polymerization
    b. resolution of fragment sizes
    c. gel casting
    d. all of the above

53. Arrested migration during gel electrophoresis could be due to:
    a. overloading
    b. depletion of electrolytes
    c. bubbles
    d. none of the above

54. Sequence amplification reactions include all of the following ecxept:
    a. PCR
    b. LCR
    c. branched DNA
    d. NASBA

55. One cycle of a polymerase chain reaction (PCR) includes:
    a. denaturation, digestion, detection
    b. denaturation, annealing, extension
    c. digestion, annealing, extension
    d. denaturation, annealing, labeling

56. All of the following are included in a PCR amplification except:
    a. thermostable polymerase
    b. target DNA
    c. amplimers
    d. amplicons

57. Annealing temperatures for the PCR range:
    a. 90–95 °C
    b. 50–60 °C
    c. 70–75 °C
    d. 30–40 °C

58. The ligase chain reaction (LCR) includes:
    a. ligation of random oligonucleotides
    b. digestion of amplified products
    c. ligation of adjacent primer pairs
    d. isothermal amplification conditions

59. The blank control in a PCR assay contains all of the following except:
    a. polymerase
    b. primers
    c. target DNA
    d. dNTPs

60. Which PCR control is used to test for specificity?
    a. blank
    b. positive
    c. negative
    d. internal housekeeping gene

61. PCR contamination control can occur by:
    a. common pipettors
    b. use of uracil-N-glycosylase
    c. washes in water baths
    d. performing all steps in one area

62. Hybrid capture technology is:
    a. a synthetic chain reaction
    b. a signal amplification reaction
    c. composed of four probes
    d. all of the above

63. RT-PCR involves all of the following except:
    a. DNA isolation
    b. reverse transcription
    c. PCR amplification
    d. product analysis

64. Nested PCR increases:
    a. the length of amplicon
    b. the specificity of reaction
    c. the stability of polymerases
    d. none of the above

65. Reverse transcriptase:
    a. amplifies target sequences
    b. results in truncated protein
    c. creates cDNA
    d. targets primary RNA transcripts

66. Primer options for RT-PCR include all of the following except:
    a. oligo (dT)
    b. random hexamers
    c. sequence specific primers
    d. oligo (dA)

67. All of the following are sexually transmitted diseases except:
    a. Chlamydia pneumoniae
    b. Neisseria gonorrhoeae
    c. HIV-1
    d. Treponema pallidum

68. The clinical symptoms of a Chlamydia infection include:
    a. salpingomas
    b. fertility
    c. urethritis
    d. tendinitis

69. The LCX Chlamydia assay targets:
    a. an organism-specific gene
    b. a host cell gene
    c. a cryptic plasmid
    d. a polymorphic sequence

70. TMA most commonly resembles which technology?
    a. NASBA
    b. SDA
    c. HCA
    d. LCR

71. Which is true for PCR?
    a. it is slower than Southern blotting
    b. it is more sensitive than Southern blotting
    c. it utilizes a single temperature
    d. it results in fragments >30 kb

72. LCR differs from PCR in that it:
    a. utilizes a single enzyme
    b. is an isothermal reaction
    c. cannot detect point mutations
    d. ligates detection probes

73. DNA is extracted from 4 mL of whole blood and resuspended in 100 µL of hydration buffer; 1 µL of this DNA is added to 999 µL of water for absorbance spectrophotometry. If the A260 is 2.0, the concentration of your DNA sample will be:
    a. 50 µg/uL
    b. 75 µg/mL
    c. 100 µg/uL
    d. 50 µg/mL

74. Which type of technology is SDA:
    a. sequence amplification
    b. signal amplification
    c. cloning
    d. electrophoretic

75. Cervical cancer is:
    a. the second most common malignancy in women
    b. the first tumor recognized as having a viral origin
    c. highly treatable and/or preventable
    d. all of the above

76. Risk factors for cervical cancer include:
    a. sexual behavior
    b. HPV type
    c. parity
    d. all of the above

77. ASCUS stands for:
    a. atypical squamous cells of uncommon source
    b. atypical squamous cells of undetermined significance
    c. abnormal squamous cells of unknown source
    d. none of the above

78. The hybrid capture assay to determine HPV type uses:
    a. individual probes
    b. two cocktails of probes
    c. DNA sequencing
    d. PCR amplification

79. HCA HPV typing is based on detection of:
    a. RNA:DNA hybrids
    b. RNA:RNA hybrids
    c. DNA:DNA hybrids
    d. none of the above

80. Direct detection of microbial pathogens by PCR analysis involves:
    a. restriction enzyme digestion
    b. fragment sizing
    c. DNA sequencing
    d. heteroduplex analysis

81. End labeling of probes:
    a. occurs at the 3'-phosphate
    b. requires a 5'-OH
    c. utilizes a polymerase
    d. none of the above

82. DEIA technology requires:
    a. DNA:DNA hybrid formation
    b. anti-RNA antibody
    c. antibody-coated wells
    d. all of the above

83. If a gene sequence is known but the mutation spectrum for that gene is unknown, you could use which technology to provide significant information?
    a. HCA
    b. PCR followed by restriction digestion
    c. SSCP
    d. ASO probes

342

84. Heteroduplex analysis requires:
    a. ssDNA
    b. agarose gel electrophoresis
    c. proper reannealing
    d. quick cooling

85. Linkage analysis and high throughput genomic screening can be used when:
    a. the gene sequence is unknown
    b. the mutation spectrum of a gene is unknown
    c. the number of mutations is too large to screen by conventional methods
    d. all of the above

86. Amplicon contamination can be prevented by all of the following except:
    a. physical barriers
    b. negative pressure rooms
    c. psoralen baths/washes
    d. UV light exposure

87. Detection in the automated ligase chain reaction is based upon all of the following except:
    a. capture haptens
    b. detection haptens
    c. unligated probe
    d. microparticle beads

Questions 88–90 refer to the following photograph of a PCR/RFLP polyacrylamide gel electrophoresis:

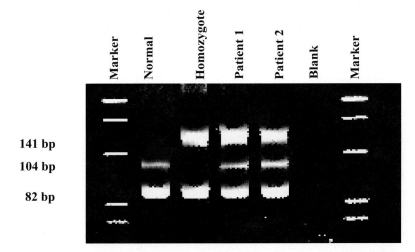

88. Given the normal and homozygous patterns for this gene mutation, what can be said about the two patient specimens?
    a. they contain a normal banding pattern
    b. they contain a homozygous banding pattern
    c. no conclusive result can be made from this gel
    d. none of the above

89. The molecular size markers are included to:
    a. accurately size fragments in patient samples
    b. monitor migration of nucleic acids
    c. control for abnormal migration or smiling
    d. all of the above

90. In this case, the mutation:
    a. destroys a restriction recognition site
    b. creates a restriction recognition site
    c. destroys a primer annealing site
    d. deletes a splice site

For questions 91–93:

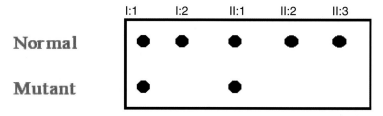

91. This dot blot was hybridized with an ASO probe specific for an autosomal recessive disease causing mutation. From the data shown, individual I:1 is a carrier for this mutation. Who else in this family carries this same abnormality?
    a. I:2 and I:3
    b. I:2 and II:1
    c. II:1 only
    d. all members of this family

92. From a family pedigree, individual II:1 is affected with the disease, yet the dot blot indicates that she is a carrier for the mutation. How do you explain this?
    a. a second mutation in the disease gene
    b. a case of non-paternity
    c. the occurrence of a genetic crossover event
    d. none of the above

93. The normal ASO probe recognizes:
    a. the normal gene sequence
    b. the normal allele sequence
    c. the intron/exon border
    d. all PCR-mplified products

94. Known mutations in an amplified PCR product may be detected by:
    a. DNA sequencing
    b. ASO probe hybridization
    c. restriction enzyme digestion
    d. all of the above

95. If you analyze a PCR product by restriction enzyme digestion and find that a patient sample has a band of lower molecular size than the normal control, you conclude that:
    a. no change in sequence is present
    b. the restriction site is lost due to mutation
    c. the restriction site is gained due to mutation
    d. the normal control is contaminated

96. A reverse dot blot utilizes what as the probe?
    a. ASO probes
    b. amplicons
    c. conjugated enzymes
    d. none of the above

97. If someone has a normal and mutant banding pattern, they are said to be:
    a. heterozygous
    b. compound homozygous
    c. homozygous
    d. wild type

98. SSCP analysis depends on:
    a. secondary structure
    b. reannealing
    c. hybridization conditions
    d. none of the above

99. In heteroduplex analysis, the heteroduplex and normal fragments are:
    a. the same sequence
    b. the same size
    c. different by >5 bases
    d. from the same PCR reaction

100. For reverse dot blots, what is labeled for detection?
    a. ASO probes
    b. PCR products
    c. the nylon membrane
    d. none of the above

101. The coding sequences of a gene are known as:
    a. exons
    b. introns
    c. splice sites
    d. frameshifts

102. A change in DNA sequence from a adenine to a thymine nucleotide is known as:
    a. transition
    b. transversion
    c. nonsense
    d. none of the above

103. The correct steps involved in Southern blot analysis include:
     a. DNA extraction > electrophoresis > amplification > transfer > hybridization
     b. Restriction digestion > extraction > electrophoresis > hybridization > transfer
     c. DNA extraction > restriction digestion > amplification > electrophoresis > hybridization
     d. DNA extraction > restriction digestion > electrophoresis > transfer > hybridization

104. Restriction endonucleases are characterized by all of the following except:
     a. bacterial enzymes that recognize DNA sequences 4 to 6 bp in length.
     b. mutations can create or destroy recognition sequences.
     c. digestion of genomic DNA results in 10–100 specific fragments.
     d. one unit of enzyme is the amount required to digest 1 μg DNA in 1 hour.

105. Knowing the charge of the DNA molecule, it migrates to the:
     a. positive cathode
     b. positive anode
     c. negative cathode
     d. negative anode

106. During the transfer of DNA for Southern blotting, larger fragments of DNA:
     a. transfer more quickly than smaller fragments
     b. transfer more efficiently than smaller fragments of DNA
     c. transfer more slowly than smaller fragments
     d. require amplification to aid in transfer

107. After transfer, all of the following are appropriate except:
     a. visualizing the gel for transfer efficiency
     b. baking the membrane to fix DNA
     c. UV crosslinking DNA to the membrane
     d. treating the membrane with a weak acid to fix DNA

108. Failure to detect a signal on a Southern blot may be due to:
     a. incomplete digestion of DNA
     b. increased stringency of post-hybridization washes
     c. improper probe labeling
     d. all of the above

109. Nucleic acid hybridization is dependent on all of the following except:
     a. temperature
     b. concentration of agarose
     c. nucleic acid sequence
     d. salt concentration

110. Random prime labeling of probes involves:
     a. utilization of random nanomers or hexamers
     b. E. coli DNA polI
     c. Dnase I
     d. none of the above

111. Plasmid DNA is:
    a. integrated into the host cell DNA
    b. complexed to histone proteins
    c. replicated by host cell enzymes
    d. commonly found in eukaryotes

112. dsDNA can be made single-stranded by increasing the temperature of the reaction or by:
    a. acidic pH
    b. neutral pH
    c. alkaline pH
    d. physiologic pH

113. DNA illuminated with ultraviolet light fluoresces due to which intercalating agent?
    a. ethidium fluoride
    b. ethidium bromide
    c. psoralen
    d. thymidine dimer

114. Restriction endonucleases recognize specific:
    a. methylation patterns
    b. trinucleotide repeats
    c. palindromic DNA sequences
    d. DNA-damaged sites

115. Cloning vectors contain all of the following except:
    a. origins of replication
    b. restriction endonuclease recognition sites
    c. antibiotic resistance genes
    d. intronic sequences

116. Stringency refers to:
    a. control of specificity of hybridization
    b. annealing of amplicons
    c. ultraviolet detection of PCR products
    d. a cruel lab director

117. A stringent hybridization for Southern blotting would include:
    a. low temperature, high salt concentration
    b. high temperature, high salt concentration
    c. high temperature, low salt concentration
    d. low temperature, low salt concentration

118. All of the following are detection methods used for probe detection except:
    a. isotopic labels
    b. enzymatic detection
    c lumiphores
    d. ethidium bromide

119. DNA sequencing based upon dideoxyribose chemistry is referred to as:
    a. Maxam-Gilbert sequencing
    b. chemical sequencing
    c. sanger sequencing
    d. manual sequencing

120. If a plasmid is 2.9 kb in size and your cloned insert is 1.2 kb in size, the size of the final isolated plasmid vector after infecting bacteria is:
    a. 2.9 kb
    b. 1.2 kb
    c. 4.1 kb
    d. 1.7 kb

121. Prehybridization solutions may contain all of the following except:
    a. casein
    b. BSA
    c. salmon sperm DNA
    d. Nick-translated probe

122. If a deletion occurs within a gene, this will be detected by Southern blot as:
    a no hybridization signal
    b. two bands with a single digest
    c. a larger size fragment than normal
    d. none of the above

123. Given the location of two invariant restriction cut sites and the probe, a mutation that creates another restriction site would result in:
    a. no amplification
    b. smaller fragment in the mutant than in the normal
    c. larger fragment in the mutant than in the normal
    d. no signal detection

124. The diagnosis of lymphoma includes all of the following except:
    a. immunopathology
    b. electron microscopy
    c. molecular genetics
    d. histochemistry

125. Maturation of a pro-thymocyte results in:
    a. a plasma cell
    b. RBC
    c. a T-cell
    d. a B-cell

126. Bcl-1 is most commonly translocated in:
    a. T-cell lymphoma
    b. Mantle cell lymphoma
    c. follicular lymphoma
    d. Hodgkin's disease

127. Immunoglobulin and T-cell receptors are:
    a. structurally similar
    b. heterodimer proteins
    c. composed of variable and constant regions
    d. all of the above

128. In addition to DNA recombination events, immune diversity can be accomplished by:
    a. germ line mutations
    b. somatic mutations
    c. apoptosis
    d. large intervening sequences

129. Clonality refers to:
    a. cells derived from a single precursor cell
    b. cells containing a specific plasmid sequence
    c. cells dividing at the same rate
    d. a polymorphic cell population

130. Applications of molecular testing to hematopathology include all of the following except:
    a. confirmation of diagnosis
    b. monitoring minimal residual disease
    c. therapeutic drug monitoring
    d. evaluation of patients after bone marrow transplant

131. Follicular center cell lymphomas are characterized by:
    a. t(14;17)
    b. bcl-2 translocation
    c. bcl-1 translocation
    d. t(11;14)

132. Disorders of lymphoid cells that result in neoplasia represent:
    a. apoptotic B- or T-cells
    b. cells arrested at various stages of development
    c. cells at the G2/M checkpoint
    d. none of the above

133. During a Southern blot transfer analysis, how much DNA is required per lane to detect a gene rearrangement?
    a. 1 μg
    b. 5 μg
    c. 10 μg
    d. 50 μg

134. In the analysis of gene rearrangements for hematologic malignancies, genomic DNA is:
    a. digested with three different enzymes
    b. hybridized with consensus sequence probes
    c. compared to a germline control DNA
    d. all of the above

135. This form of analysis is the "gold standard" for detection of clonal populations of cells that are represented by novel banding patterns. Novel bands include any band other than:
    a. a germline band
    b. a pseudohybridization band
    c. bands due to partial digestion
    d. all of the above

Question 136 pertains to the following Southern blot transfer analysis:

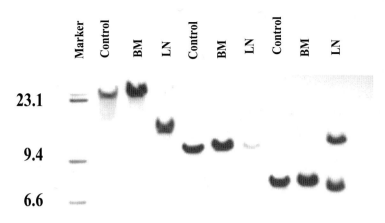

136. In the above Southern blot, a bone marrow (BM) and lymph node (LN) specimen from the samepatient are analyzed. Novel bands are identified in:
    a. both specimens
    b. only the bone marrow
    c. only the lymph node
    d. neither of the specimens

137. PCR analysis for B- and T-cell gene rearrangements:
    a. is less sensitive than Southern blot
    b. results in more false negative cases than Southern blot
    c. is more labor intense than Southern blot
    d. requires highly purified DNA

138. During PCR analysis for B-cell gene rearrangements, gel electrophoresis produces a negative result. In addition, the blank, negative and positive control all worked as expected. You can conclude:
    a. the specimen does not contain a clonal population of B-cells
    b. the specimen contains a polyclonal population of B-cells
    c. the results are indeterminate
    d. this may be a T-cell lesion

139. Sanger DNA sequencing:
    a. requires piperidine cleavage
    b. incorporates dideoxynucleotides
    c. depends upon restriction recognition sites
    d. terminates reactions by overloading dATP

140. In addition to performing direct DNA sequencing on PCR amplicons for mutation detection, which of the following techniques can be used as a screening method:
    a. Southern blot
    b. ASO probes
    c. heteroduplex analysis
    d. restriction digest

141. Advantages of FISH include all of the following except:
    a. decreased turnaround time
    b. dual detection capability
    c. rapidly dividing cells
    d. analysis of tissue heterogeneity

142. Alpha satellite probes:
    a. are used in conjunction with single copy probes
    b. are used to identify marker chromosomes
    c. can function as internal controls
    d. all of the above

Match the following tumors with their corresponding molecular marker. Place the letter in the space provided by the tumor type.

143. neuroblastoma _____   a. IgH

144. NHL, B-cell _____   b. EWS/WT1

145. DSRCT _____   c. SYT/SSX

146. synovial sarcoma _____   d. Del 1p

Match the following tumors with their corresponding treatment. Place the letter in the space provided by the tumor type.

147. neuroblastoma _____   a. adriamycin

148. PNET_____   b. dactinomycin

149. rhabdomyosarcoma _____   c. platinum

150. In detecting the most common molecular defect in neuroblastoma by FISH analysis, you wouldutilize:
    a. two single-copy probes
    b. an alpha satellite and single-copy probe
    c. a chromosome paint
    d. none of the above

Match the temperatures on the right with the best choice on the left. Each answer may be used more than once.

151. whole blood for DNA extraction _____   a. 24 °C

152. DNA storage for two years _____   b. 4 °C

153. RNA storage _____   c –20 °C

154. long-term tissue storage _____   d. –70 °C

155. Spectrophotometry can provide all of the following data except:
    a. quantity of DNA
    b. quantity of RNA
    c. quality of nucleic acid
    d. purity of nucleic acid

156. Migration rate of a macromolecule through a gel matrix during electrophoresis depends on:
    a. net charge on the molecule
    b. size of the molecule
    c. specific gel matrix
    d. all of the above

Questions 157–161 refer to the following Southern blot, whereby an invariant cut site separates the two probe regions. One blot was probed with probe A and the other with probe B.

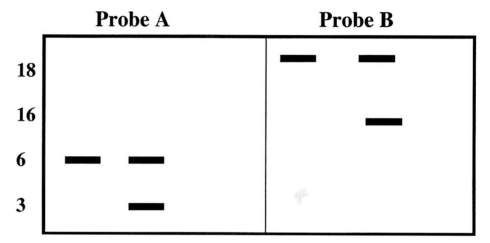

157. In this two-probe/one-restriction enzyme Southern blot, how many polymorphic cut sites are there? (Hint: Draw the schematic showing the probe and gene sequence.)
    a. one
    b. two
    c. three
    d. four

158. What is the most likely genotype of the individual in lane 1 of each blot? (Hint: Examine each probe separately.)
    a. 0,0
    b. 0,1
    c. 0,2
    d. indeterminate

159. What is the genotype of the individual in lane 2 of each blot (Hint: examine each probe separately):
    a. 0,1
    b. 1,2
    c. 0,2
    d. indeterminate

160. If lane 1 represents a father affected with an autosomal recessive disorder, what conclusions can be reached concerning this family?
    a. the mother (lane 2) is a carrier of the recessive mutation
    b. their offspring have a 50% chance of being affected
    c. the mother has a 50% chance of passing on the disease gene
    d. none of the above

161. If lane 1 represents a child with an X-linked recessive disease, what can be said about her siblings?
    a. all brothers have a 25% chance of inheriting the disease
    b. all sisters will at least be carriers of the disease
    c. all sisters will be affected with the disease
    d. one parent is an obligate carrier of the disease gene

Questions 162–165. DNA marker studies were performed for a family whose pedigree is shown below using RFLP markers closely linked to the gene for adult polycystic kidney disease (Hint: AR disorder). Determine whether or not each of the individuals have inherited the mutant gene.

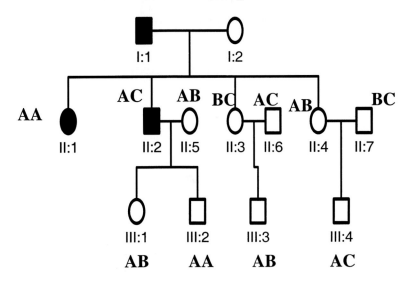

Place the appropriate letter next to the individual in question. Each answer can be used more than once.

162. individual III-1. _____   a. probably carries the APKD mutation

163. individual III-2 _____   b. probably does not carry the mutation

164. individual III-3 _____   c. cannot be determined from the given
                                       information
165. individual III-4 _____

For questions 166–171, match each term with one of the following items which best fits.

166. alleleic heterogeneity_____   a. expressed in heterozygotes

167. dominant_____   b. X-inactivation

168. expressivity _____   c. de novo

169. lyonization _____   d. same locus

170. obligate carrier _____   e. clinical heterogeneity

171. sporadic _____   f. pedigree analysis

For questions 172–174, refer to the following pedigree:

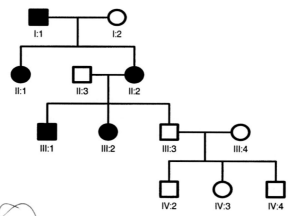

172. The mode of inheritance depicted in this family pedigree is:
    a. non-Mendelian
    b. X-linked dominant
    c. X-linked recessive
    d. autosomal recessive

173. Daughters of an affected male have what chance of being affected with the disease?
    a. 25%
    b. 33%
    c. 50%
    d. 100%

174. Affected individuals will have:
    a. an affected parent
    b. an obligate carrier parent
    c. unaffected offspring
    d. none of the above

Questions 175–178 refer to the following pedigree. The frequency of this autosomal recessive disease in the general population is 1 in 50,000.

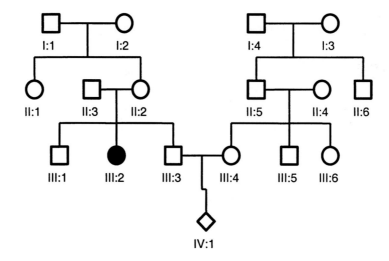

175. What is III:4's chance of carrying the mutated gene?
     a. 1/224
     b. 223/224
     c. 1/112
     d. 1/50

176. What is III:3's chance of being a carrier of the mutated gene?
     a. 1/4
     b. 1/2
     c. 2/3
     d. 1

177. What is IV:1's chance of being a carrier of the disease causing mutation?
     a. ½
     b. 1/112
     c. 1/252
     d. 1/336

178. If III:2 were to have a child, what is the chance that the child will be affected with the disease?
     a. 1/112
     b. 1/224
     c. 1/336
     d. 1/448

179. Sickle cell trait is characterized by:
     a. hematuria
     b. homozygous mutant
     c. hemolytic anemia
     d. clinical heterogeneity

180. Cystic fibrosis is characterized by:
     a. infertility
     b. lung tumors
     c. progressive kidney failure
     d. none of the above

181. The most common molecular defect in CF is:
     a. a 3-bp deletion
     b. a translocation
     c. a point mutation
     d. a rearrangement

182. BMD is characterized by:
     a. deleted protein
     b. splice site mutations
     c. truncated protein
     d. none of the above

183. Fragile X syndrome is:
     a. the most common form of hereditary mental retardation
     b. an X-linked dominant disorder
     c. due to anticipation
     d. diagnosed at birth

184. Southern blot analysis for Fragile X syndrome is:
     a. dependent upon the probe/enzyme combination used
     b. detected as a 5.2-kb and 2.8-kb banding pattern
     c. useful for identifying the active and inactive X chromosmes
     d. useful for identifying abnormal FRAX mutations

185. Hereditary hemochromatosis is due to:
     a. excessive iron overload
     b. organ dysfunction
     c. a single polymorphism
     d. quantitative phlebotomy

186. The C282Y mutation in the HFE gene can be detected by:
     a. PCR and MnlI digestion
     b. ASO probe
     c. PCR and DpnII digestion
     d. none of the above

187. The analytical sensitivity of an assay is based on:
     a. clinical outcome
     b. number of true negatives
     c. limit of detection
     d. number of false positives

188. An ASO probe will detect:
     a. a single mutation or allelic sequence
     b. several mutations in a given gene sequence
     c. X-linked mutations only
     d. all of the above

189. Malignant tumor cells have:
     a. a rapid growth rate
     b. slow cell cycle progression
     c. two acquired and one inherited mutation
     d. resulted from multiple stem cells

190. Which of the following have been shown to be involved in the development of human cancers?
     a. environmental factors
     b. radiation
     c. EBV
     d. all of the above

191. The first tumor suppressor gene to be cloned was:
     a. p53
     b. RB
     c. N-myc
     d. BRCA1

192. Mutation of a proto-oncogene results in all of the following except:
     a. gain of function
     b. decreased cell division
     c. qualitative change in gene expression
     d. dominant inheritance pattern

193. The most common oncogene to be affected in human cancer is:
    a. ras
    b. p53
    c. c-myc
    d. HER2

194. The t(8;14) translocation involves which genes?
    a. BL and IgH
    b. c-myc and IgH
    c. c-myc and ras
    d. c-myc and TCR

195. Translocations can lead to:
    a. new protein expression
    b. fusion transcripts
    c. deletion of genetic material
    d. all of the above

196. Which gene has been shown to be amplified in human cancer?
    a. c-myc
    b. N-myc
    c. BRCA1
    d. H-ras

197. p53 regulates which cell cycle checkpoint?
    a. G1/S
    b. G2/S
    c. G2/M
    d. G0/S

198. p53 functions in all of the following except:
    a. DNA repair
    b. DNA replication
    c. cell division
    d. apoptosis

199. The characteristic hallmark of human cancer is:
    a. metastatic disease
    b. abnormal cell growth and proliferation
    c clonality
    d. acquired mutations

200. DNA damage can result in a stable mutation if:
    a. DNA repair is slow
    b. the affected gene is early replicating
    c. there is deficient DNA repair
    d. all of the above

201. Telomerase activity is:
    a. absent in germline cells
    b. increased in tumor cells
    c. required for cell senescence
    d. required for deletion of telomeric sequences

202. Signs of hereditary cancer include:
    a. autosomal recessive pattern of inheritance
    b. multiple affected organs
    c. early age of onset
    d. all of the above

203. Retinoblastoma is characterized by all of the following except:
    a. hereditary component
    b. acquired component
    c. inactivation of the RAS gene
    d. de novo mutation

204. FAP is associated with:
    a. HNPCC gene mutations
    b. poor prognosis
    c. 25% frequency of p53 mutations
    d. abnormal mismatch repair

205. The Amsterdam criteria for diagnosing HNPCC include all of the following except:
    a. at least 3 affected family members
    b. at least one generation represented
    c. at least 1 individual less than 50 years of age
    d. two first degree relatives are affected

206. All of the following are true about breast cancer except:
    a. 1 in 9 women will develop breast cancer in the U.S.
    b. 5–10% of all breast cancer is hereditary
    c. family history is the best risk factor for breast cancer
    d. BRCA 1 and BRCA 2 mutations account for the majority of herediatry breast cancer

207. Which stage of breast cancer is associated with the best prognosis?
    a. stage I
    b. stage II
    c. stage III
    d. stage IV

208. The majority of Ewing's/PNET tumors have which translocation?
    a. t(8;14)
    b. t(11;22)
    c. t(15;17)
    d. t(9;12)

209. Gene amplification can be detected by:
    a. FISH
    b. dPCR
    c. Southern blot
    d. all of the above

210. The major application of molecular tests in evaluating B- and T-cell neoplasms is:
    a. establishing a prognosis
    b. determining clonality
    c. detecting translocations
    d. none of the above

211. Mantle cell lymphomas are characterized by:
    a. t(14;17)
    b. bcl-2 translocation
    c. bcl-1 translocation
    d. t(11;14)

212. T-cell clonality is determined by evaluating:
    a. immunoglobulin heavy chain gene rearrangements
    b. bcl-2 gene translocations
    c. bcr/abl
    d. T-cell receptor gene rearrangements

213. During a Southern blot transfer analysis, DNA is extracted and then:
    a. electrophoresed in agarose gels
    b. hybridized with a gene-specific probe
    c. digested with specific restriction endonucleases
    d. none of the above

214. Small clones of tumor cells in a patient that may result in relapse of disease are referred to as:
    a. minimal tumor content
    b. minimal residual disease
    c. hypodiploidy
    d. tumor burden

215. Identity testing has been performed using all of the following except:
    a. ABO typing
    b. HLA typing
    c. heteroduplex analysis
    d. RFLP analysis

216. A change in the restriction recognition site for an enzyme is:
    a. a sequence polymorphism
    b. a size polymorphism
    c. a VNTR
    d. an STR

217. All of the following are required for DNA based parentage testing except:
    a. maternal DNA
    b. child's DNA
    c. chain of custody
    d. testing documentation

218. The paternity index (PI) refers to:
    a. the probability of paternity
    b. the likelihood of a given genotype in the general population
    c. the likelihood that the matching allele is from the alleged father
    d. the factors favoring paternity

219. An alleged father is excluded as being the biological father of the child when:
    a. he does not share more than two obligate paternal alleles with the child
    b. the maternal alleles account for both childs alleles
    c. he shares one of two alleles with the child
    d. he is not recognized by the mother or child

For questions 220–222, refer to the following data:

Marker	Mother	Child	Alleged father
D3S1358	17	17,18	16,17
VWA	15,19	15,16	16,18
D16S539	10,11	11	12,13
D2S1338	17	17,20	24,25

220. The obligate maternal genotype for markers D3S1358, vWA, D16S539, and D2S1338 in this child is:
    a. 17,15,11,17
    b. 17,19,10,17
    c. 18,16,11,17
    d. indeterminate

221. The paternal obligate genotype for these same markers is:
    a. 16,16,11,24
    b. 16,18,13,25
    c. 18, 16, 11,20
    d. 17,16,13,24

222. Based on these testing results, you can conclude that:
    a. the alleged father cannot be excluded as the biological father of the child
    b. the alleged father can be excluded as the biological father of the child
    c. the results are indeterminate
    d. more markers would need to be run

For questions 223–225, refer to the following data:

Marker	Mother	Child	Alleged father
D8S1179	11,13	13,15	14,15
D21S11	28,32.2	27,32.2	27,31.2
D18S51	12,15	12,14	14,16

223. Given the following allele frequencies, calculate the paternity index for the D8S1179 marker.
    Allele 11, 0.002; allele 13, 0.654, allele 15, 0.143; allele 14, 0.234; HINT: PI=1/2q
    a. 0.76
    b. 3.50
    c. 2.14
    d. 0.143

224. If the paternity indices for markers D21S11 and D18S51 are 7.8 and 1.4, respectively, the CPI would be:
    a. 12.70
    b. 23.37
    c. 38.22
    d. 8.30

225. The resulting CPP would be:
    a. 92.02%
    b. 95.90%
    c. 97.45%
    d. 89.25%

Answers

1. d	35. c	69. a	103. d
2. b	36. a	70. a	104. c
3. d	37. a	71. b	105. b
4. c	38. c	72. d	106. c
5. c	39. c	73. c	107. d
6. e	40. b	74. b	108. d
7. a	41. a	75. d	109. b
8. d	42. e	76. d	110. a
9. b	43. c	77. b	111. a
10. c	44. d	78. b	112. c
11. b	45. b	79. c	113. b
12. a	46. a	80. a	114. c
13. c	47. c	81. b	115. d
14. b	48. c	82. c	116. a
15. b	49. a	83. a	117. c
16. a	50. b	84. b	118. d
17. b	51. d	85. d	119. c
18. a	52. d	86. c	120. c
19. b	53. c	87. c	121. d
20. a	54. c	88. d	122. a
21. d	55. b	89. d	123. b
22. b	56. d	90. a	124. b
23. b	57. b	91. c	125. c
24. b	58. c	92. a	126. b
25. c	59. c	93. b	127. d
26. d	60. c	94. d	128. a
27. c	61. b	95. c	129. a
28. b	62. b	96. b	130. c
29. c	63. a	97. a	131. b
30. d	64. b	98. a	132. b
31. d	65. c	99. b	133. c
32. a	66. d	100. b	134. d
33. b	67. a	101. a	135. d
34. a	68. c	102. b	136. c

Molecular Diagnostics

—

—

—

137. b	160. d	183. a	206. b
138. a	161. b	184. a	207. a
139. b	162. a	185. a	208. b
140. c	163. a	186. b	209. d
141. c	164. b	187. c	210. b
142. d	165. a	188. a	211. c
143. d	166. d	189. a	212. d
144. a	167. a	190. d	213. c
145. b	168. e	191. b	214. b
146. c	169. b	192. b	215. c
147. b	170. f	193. a	216. a
148. c	171. c	194. b	217. a
149. a	172. b	195. d	218. c
150. b	173. d	196. b	219. a
151. a	174. a	197. a	220. a
152. b	175. d	198. c	221. c
153. a	176. b	199. b	222. b
154. d	177. b	200. d	223. c
155. b	178. b	201. b	224. b
156. d	179. d	202. d	225. b
157. b	180. a	203. c	
158. a	181. a	204. b	
159. b	182. c	205. b	